Five Easy Steps
to Prevent Falls

*The Comprehensive Guide to
Keeping Patients of All Ages Safe*

Deanna Gray-Miceli, PhD, GNP-BC, FAANP, FAAN

AMERICAN NURSES ASSOCIATION
2014

American Nurses Association
8515 Georgia Avenue, Suite 400
Silver Spring, MD 20910-3492
1-800-274-4ANA
www.NursingWorld.org

Published by the Nursing Knowledge Center
www.nursingknowledgecenter.org

The American Nurses Association (ANA) is the only full-service professional organization representing the interests of the nation's 3.1 million registered nurses through its constituent/state nurses associations and its organizational affiliates. The ANA advances the nursing profession by fostering high standards of nursing practice, promoting the rights of nurses in the workplace, projecting a positive and realistic view of nursing, and by lobbying the Congress and regulatory agencies on healthcare issues affecting nurses and the public.

978-1-55810-567-6   SAN: 851-3481   11/2015R
First printing: September 2014.   Second printing: November 2015.

To my dear daughter and husband,
whose support has been timely and tremendous.

Contents

About the Author

Deanna Gray-Miceli, PhD, GNP-BC, FAANP, FAAN is Assistant Professor at Rutgers University, School of Nursing, Newark, New Jersey; and Adjunct Assistant Professor, University of Pennsylvania, School of Nursing. She is a clinical scholar and national falls prevention expert whose innovation has centered on developing and testing a comprehensive post-fall assessment for practicing RNs called the Post-Fall Index™ (PFI). Proven to be effective in reducing falls, the PFI™ provides professional nurses with a decision support tool used for determining why a fall occurred in the first place. Dr. Gray-Miceli's 30-plus year career as an advanced practice gerontological nurse practitioner has centered on the care of the vulnerable, frail elderly in long-term care. In the 1990s, she founded and directed one of the first nurse-driven, interdisciplinary fall prevention programs in the country, the Fall Assessment and Prevention Program, housed at the University of Medicine and Dentistry of New Jersey Center for Aging.

Dr. Gray-Miceli has also served as Project Director to New York University for the development of the educational blueprint and curricula leading to the nationally acclaimed, Geriatric Nursing Education Consortium (GNEC), sponsored by the American Association of Colleges of Nursing and the John Hartford Institute for Geriatric Nursing.

She is an invited consultant for the development of state-led falls prevention initiatives across the continuum of care in New Jersey. This includes serving as co-chair of the Falls Committee of the UMDNJ-School of Public Health and Injury Prevention Workgroup of the New Jersey Department of Health, and co-representative to that state's National Council on Aging Falls Free Task Force.

Since 2012, she has served as the Evidence-Based Practice (EBP) Falls co-leader to the National Training and Coordination Collaborative (NTACC), which oversees programs developed by HRSA-funded Geriatric Education Centers (GEC). She also provides consultation to long-term care facilities on falls prevention and reduction, as well as a consultative fall prevention practice.

Dr. Gray-Miceli received her BSN from Farleigh Dickinson University, MSN from the University of Pennsylvania, and PhD from Widener University. She is a Distinguished Alumni, Fairleigh Dickinson University, Henry P. Becton School of Nursing and Allied Health, Metropolitan Campus, Teaneck, NJ.

Dr. Gray-Miceli has been a John A. Hartford Post-Doctoral Scholar at the University of Pennsylvania, a Fellow of the Gerontological Society of America, a Fellow of the American Academy of Nurse Practitioners; and a Fellow of the American Academy of Nursing and a Scholar, National Institute of Aging.

Preface: Why This Book?

After many years of spending long hours walking up and down corridors of hospital and nursing home units caring for frail older adults, most of whom were falling frequently, I wondered to myself, "What is going on?" Despite my best efforts to reduce falls, patients were still falling. Is it disease? Environment? Functional impairment? Medication side effects? None of these, or all of these? The pursuit of answers to these questions has spurred my research and clinical scholarship, and is the origin of my work, which is centered on determining factors responsible for the fall using patient and provider perspectives. Getting to the "why" of the fall is rooted in a comprehensive post-fall assessment.

All of the possible multifactorial causal event factors for falls were swirling through my head. In the 1980s when I started out, we simply provided good nursing care. There were no protocols, no national guidelines, no evidenced-based practices, just good nursing care, which was its own "best practice." With each and every patient encounter, I asked with intrigue, "Tell me what happened, what you were doing, and what we can do to reduce your falls."

As the years passed, I accumulated a collection of vivid stories and accounts of patient falls, many of which painted similar pictures. I decided to use these unwritten, vivid experiences for patient betterment. So I enrolled in doctoral course work, ultimately conducting my dissertation around the lived experiences and meaning of serious falls to older adults living independently in the community. Never did I imagine what I would hear, and what interpretive analysis would later reveal.

Marion, a retired pediatric nurse practitioner in her late 80s, grabbed me by my lab coat and remarked, "Please! Find out *why* I am falling!" 92-year-old Andrianne said, "Well you know... Deanna... after the fall, we would walk to the dining room, and I would hold my husband's arm, not just in affection, but you know... but in desperation and fear, 'Hold me up so I don't fall again!'"

Nurses in every part of their journey, caring for patients of all ages, and in all practice settings hear similar stories and are witness to the patient's perspective. The patient's perspective is half the story; the other half is what the provider thinks and does about the fall. As a qualitative researcher and nurse practitioner guided by humanistic care, patient stories and dissertation research have shaped my understanding about falls and injury prevention which I share in this book.

Influenced by the best teams of colleagues in academic geriatrics and geriatric nursing, public health, and biostatistics and epidemiology at the University of Pennsylvania, I discovered the essence of what nurses can be empowered to do should they be provided with the right clinical assessment tools to inform their decisions about fall care so they too can begin to answer the question of why the fall happened in the first place. My career-changing focus in patient-centered research developed as a result of receiving the prestigious John A. Hartford Post-Doctoral Scholarship. Along with a team of mentors, I was able to concentrate on research related to the reduction of falls by means of developing and validating a nurse-driven, patient-centered comprehensive post-fall assessment tool, the Post-Fall Index (PFI), capable of assisting nurses in long-term care as a clinical decision support tool. A wonderful opportunity was then developed to study the effects of the PFI on total and recurrent falls with a cohort of older adults in long-term care. This was done with support and funding from the Academic Geriatric Long-Term Care Award, Division of Geriatric Medicine at the University of Pennsylvania. The study found that the PFI reduced falls significantly. In follow-up years, additional secondary analyses of the falls dataset obtained in this study have been conducted. Many important "Ah ha!" moments from this research are echoed in this book based on particular pieces of our work. Two of these pieces of work directly impacting patient care and nursing practice are the findings related to the care of patients with orthostatic hypotension and findings regarding ambulatory older adults residing in assisted living who incur post-fall head injuries.

The purpose of this book is to provide all practicing nurses with practical methods for identifying fall and injury risks as well as their underlying causes by means of performing the best assessment possible utilizing five easy steps. Fall assessment, fall reduction and injury prevention are possible given the right knowledge, clinical skills and appropriate assessment tools. Fall and injury prevention is never one-sided—it involves developing a shared perspective between patient and provider and determining a mutually acceptable plan of care that is humanistic, holistic and above all, person-centered.

As a national falls-prevention expert, my contribution to nursing science is to empower other nurses to broaden their vision, to understand the falling victims' perspectives, and to actively listen to patients' experiences so that various perspectives of the phenomena of a fall may be revealed and used to formulate specific care plans for falls prevention.

I drew heavily from the role of nurses in public health, my recollections of anecdotal and patient reports, evidence-based research findings, recollections from nurses in practice, and from a large library of fall photographs I have accrued over the years. Many of these fall photographs I have used to teach nurses and patients alike. I have also drawn on the collective works from professional societies such as the evidence-based recommendations from the American Geriatrics Society Guidelines for Falls Prevention, the John A. Hartford Institute for Geriatric Nursing at NYU, and the John A. Hartford Foundation Center of Geriatric Nursing Excellence (HCGNE) at the University of Iowa's College of Nursing.

Other important works referenced in this book are drawn from public health sources such as the Center for Disease Control, National Center for Injury Prevention and Control, the National Patient Safety Commission, the Institute for Healthcare Improvement and the VISN 8 Patient Safety Center of Inquiry, Veteran's Administration, the American Nurses Association, the National Quality Forum, and the Joint Commission on Accreditation of Hospital Associations.

I was privileged to have some excellent reviewers from different professional backgrounds who read earlier drafts of this book and whose comments, suggestions, and insights proved invaluable to me. They are: Pat Quigley, PhD, MPH, ARNP, CRRN, FAAN, FAANP, Associate Director, VISN 8 Patient Safety Center of Inquiry, a renowned researcher and contributor to clinical practice innovations in patient safety (particularly in falls prevention), nursing, and rehabilitation activities at the national level... Dee Kumpar, MBA, BSN, RN, CSPHP, developer of SPHM programs for Kaiser Permanente and Ascension Health, a member of the Board of Directors of the Association of Safe Patient Handling Professionals, and a member of the workgroup that developed and wrote ANA's SPHM National Interprofessional Standards... Michelle Feil MSN, RN, Senior Patient Safety Analyst, Pennsylvania Patient Safety Authority and ECRI Institute... Jaime Dawson, MPH, Senior Policy Analyst of ANA's Department of Nursing Practice and Work Environment, and staff contributor to the development of ANA's SPHM Standards.

My source of inspiration, however, for my work and this topic will always be the unanswered question of *Why did the fall occur*? This question of *why* is the reason the Post-Fall Index was first developed as a comprehensive assessment tool and an index to uncover the underlying likely cause of an older adult's fall. It is also the guiding reason which supports healthcare professionals' assessment of the patient.

As you will see when you flip through the photographs and read the narrative, a vast amount of material drives my passion to not only prevent falls, but also to reduce errors in post-fall treatment. That passion for falls prevention developed not only from patient accounts and research findings about falls across all age groups but also from several significant events involving family members' declines in health and mobility following a fracture-related fall.

Acknowledgments

The pages in this book reflect the assimilated voices, events, and inspirations bestowed to me through patients, friends, colleagues, and family. I cherish these shared experiences and collectively they have helped to facilitate my work accomplished in this book. I dedicate this book to the following individuals:

My dear daughter and husband, whose support has been timely and tremendous. I could not have done it without all of your support and love: you endured my endless hours of typing and trips to facilities to make this book whole. I am indebted to your pitching in, magnificent culinary skills, and family spirit while also carrying a very heavy load as high school scholar, musician, and much more.

To my many relatives who incurred unexpected and unexplained falls, some of which heralded the beginning of a spiraling decline. Yet, still we have many unanswered questions of "why"?

Among those seeking answers are a dedicated prestigious informal team of colleagues, mentors, and friends who have stood by me for many years, producing many publications, scientific presentations, and scholarly research. Thank you for graciously allowing me to indoctrinate your world of medicine, biostatistics, public health, epidemiology, and psychology with older adult falls and their prevention. I would like to especially acknowledge Drs. Jerry Johnson, MD, Sarah Ratcliffe, PhD, Tom Zanna, and Giles Crane MPH, ASA for their steadfast support, guidance, mentorship, and friendship over the years. The input from a state's perspective in public health from my colleagues, Dr. Martin Zanna, Marian Passananate, and Bill Haplerin have more clearly defined what needs to be done in our society for public good. As falls prevention involves such a broad, supportive interdisciplinary team, every day I value the contribution from the physical sciences such as engineering. A big thank you to Dr. Norm Badler for helping me connect the angles, so to speak.

Falls prevention policy change is needed for all ages. I am thankful to those academic geriatric nursing faculty whose leadership has embraced my work and helped me to leverage an important public health platform for older adults. Mentorship by Neville Strumpf, Mathy Mezey, and Taylor Harden has helped me journey down this road over many years.

In 2002, The John A. Hartford Foundation embraced, funded, and nurtured my work as a clinical scholar, which allowed me not only to produce important, scholarly work, but to work closely and develop relationships with similarly minded colleagues in nursing and falls prevention.

I could not have done this book without the generous support and time from Dr. Pat Quigley. Thank you for being such a spectacular role model, colleague, and friend! Pat ... You do it all so effortlessly, from bedside clinical research in falls and injury protection to translational science with teams of followers and a practice in falls prevention. The tremendous editorial support and technical advice of the ANA publications development production team, headed by Eric Wurzbacher, has allowed me to not fall behind in developing the content for this book.

And lastly, to all of the older adult patients who have been victim to falls. I am fortunate to have a falls prevention practice, which keeps me grounded to the world of practice and the lives touched, altered and in some cases devastated by falls. Your countless experiences will continue to be the inspiration and motivation which have prompted writing of this book. Let's hope one day soon, a patient's wish to find out why their unexplained falls occurred is answered. Until then, I hope this book sets in motion the needed practice change in the way we approach, define, plan and prevent falls and injuries for all patients in all healthcare settings. In particular, the 19 unforgettable patients and their families who participated in my qualitative dissertation research and spurred my journey in falls prevention, thank you for sharing your wisdom and world views. Although it was many years ago, your experiences still ring true in the eyes of other older adults who fall.

—Deanna Gray-Miceli

Introduction: What You Can Do with This Book

Five Easy Steps to Prevent Falls is a must-have, comprehensive, user-friendly, "how-to" text for all practicing nurses working in hospitals, long-term care or the community working with adult and older adult populations. Nurses will learn, based on current fall theory and epidemiology, how patients define falls, and the *what, when, where* and most importantly, the *why* of the fall. Emphasis is placed on the needs of the older adult. Colored photographs highlight high-risk areas for falls and injury potential along with educational tips on how nurses can prevent falls and teach patients to do so as well.

This book is brimming with evidence-based practice suggestions related to the primary and secondary prevention of falls and injuries, including national and international web-based resources, clinical practice guidelines, clinical tips, and special considerations for circumstances where falling patients are more likely. Throughout the book, patient safety, quality of care and patient-centeredness are emphasized. There is a strong focus on public health and its principles, which guide the falls-prevention content contained in this book. Although patients encountered in many settings are considered "residents" or clients, this book uses the terminology client to refer to the patient who has a medical encounter with the nurse. Readers do not need prior knowledge of fall theory or epidemiology: case points are presented to readers throughout the text on fall facts and statistics from national data sources, such as the Centers for Disease Control and Injury Prevention, the National Patient Safety Commission, the American Nurses Association, the National Quality Forum, and the Joint Commission on Accreditation of Hospital Associations.

This book is geared toward registered nursing professionals and students in undergraduate and graduate nursing, medical and public health schools, and professionals in physical and occupational therapy and aims to familiarize these groups with the basics of falls and injury prevention. Readers will learn how to assess at-risk patients and those who have recently fallen. This text presents various tried-and-true techniques, assessment tools and teaching strategies. *Five Easy Steps to Prevent Falls* content is comprised of the following:

- Foundational information on falls, including a unique public health perspective on this topic
- Step 1, a fall-focused health history
- Step 2, a fall-focused physical assessment
- Step 3, identifying common environmental hazards and modifying the environment for patient safety
- Step 4, effective communication for falls prevention
- Step 5, patient education for falls prevention.

Readers will be able to:

- Apply the public health model to inform, educate and empower nurses and other healthcare professionals working with patient populations at risk for falls or who have fallen;
- Determine the *what, when, where*, and *why* of falls based on current science;
- Identify key symptoms associated with preventable falls and medical emergencies;
- Learn how to safely administer basic tests of gait and balance;
- Learn when to refer patients to specialists and physical therapists;
- Increase knowledge of useful screening measures for falls and injury and practice implications;
- Recognize and assess patients for orthostatic hypotension;
- Identify early signs of post-fall head injury and other types of injury;
- Visualize first-hand the high-risk environmental hazards causing falls and how to make the environment safe for patients;
- Learn the best methods to communicate the essential aspects of fall assessment, management and overall fall care;
- Learn methods to promote patient safety and quality of care across multiple healthcare providers and settings;
- Learn about the highly acclaimed National Patient Safety Models for communication: Team STEPPS: SBAR, Hand-offs, Huddle, HEAR ME, etc.; and
- Gain insight on teaching techniques to optimize patient skill about falls prevention.

A Public Health Perspective and Background Information on Falls and Falls Prevention

A Public Health Approach to Falls and Fall-Related Injury Prevention

The Centers for Disease Control and Prevention's mission for all of public health is clearly stated in the tagline "CDC 24/7: Saving lives. Protecting People" (IOM, 1988). Among its many purposes, public health protects against environmental hazards, prevents injuries, assures the quality and accessibility of services and promotes and encourages healthy behaviors.

Core functions of public health include three broad domains: assessment, policy development and public assurance. In the context of these core functions are the Ten Essential Public Health Services, seven of which provide a framework for this book (CDC, 2014):

1. Monitor health status to identify and solve community problems;
2. Diagnose and investigate health problems and health in the community;
3. Inform, educate and empower people;
4. Develop policies and plans that support individual and community health efforts;
5. Link people to needed personal health services and provide care;
6. Assure a competent public and personal healthcare workforce;
7. Evaluate effectiveness, accessibility, and quality of programs and population-based health services.

Upon completion of *Five Easy Steps to Prevent Falls*, readers will be knowledgeable to work collaboratively with others to develop action plans centered on the three remaining essential public health services:

- ► Mobilize community partnerships and action to identify and solve health problems related to falls prevention,
- ► Enforce laws and regulations that protect health and ensure safety, and
- ► Research new insights and innovative solutions to health problems related to falls and their prevention.

The overall purpose of this book is reflected in the sixth Essential Public Health Service function listed above: "to assure a competent public and personal healthcare workforce" (2014). Moreover, these seven of the Ten Essential Public Health Services provide a broad framework for specific content and educational objectives discussed in each chapter of *Five Easy Steps to Prevent Falls*. Because *Five Easy Steps to Prevent Falls* is concerned with individual-level assessment by nurses, quality and safety for patients who fall, and safety among the healthcare nursing workforce, equally important objectives are referenced within *Five Easy Steps to Prevent Falls* with respect to the following areas:

- ► Culture of safety
- ► Healthcare worker safety
- ► Safe patient handling and mobility (SPHM), including the interprofessional national standards for SPHM developed by the American Nurses Association (ANA, 2013)
- ► Adequate staffing (ANA, 2012)

Significance of Falls in America

Falls and injury prevention are public health priorities in the United States across all age groups, from infants and children to older adults over age 85. Falls have no geographic boundary, a fact illustrated by the landscape of unintentional injury deaths and non-fatal injuries due to falls from the northern to southern regions and from the eastern to western coastline (see Figure 1).

Falls and fall-related injuries affect men and women of all races. Evidence shows there is a widespread distribution of falls throughout the United States. Based on the most current data (1999–2010) from the Centers for Disease Control and Prevention (CDC), for all age groups combined (less than 1 year through 85 and older), death due to falls ranks #3 nationwide. Current

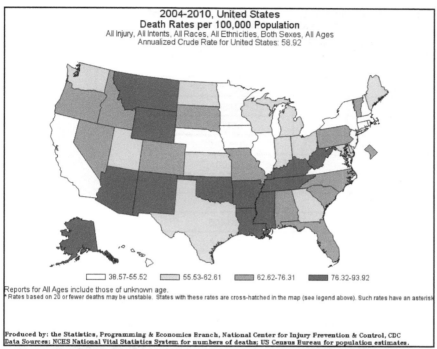

2004-2010, United States
Death Rates per 100,000 Population
All Injury, All Intents, All Races, All Ethnicities, Both Sexes, All Ages
Annualized Crude Rate for United States: 58.92

38.57-55.52   55.53-62.61   62.62-76.31   76.32-93.92

Reports for All Ages include those of unknown age.
* Rates based on 20 or fewer deaths may be unstable. States with these rates are cross-hatched in the map (see legend above). Such rates have an asterisk

Produced by: the Statistics, Programming & Economics Branch, National Center for Injury Prevention & Control, CDC
Data Sources: NCHS National Vital Statistics System for numbers of deaths; US Census Bureau for population estimates.

Figure 1. U.S. falls-related injury deaths.

rankings place deaths due to falls as the number one cause of injury-related deaths among 65–74 year-olds, 75–84 year-olds, and those 85+ (Table 1). Fall deaths ranked #3 among persons 35–64 years of age. In 2012, non-fatal falls for all ages combined ranked #1 in cause of injury and affected more than 7 million Americans (CDC, n.d. 1). In these instances, the non-fatal fall results in an emergency room visit, hospitalization or transfer to a facility for care (Table 2).

The population level data provided in Tables 1 and 2 provide not only information about various populations who fall, but also educational resources (CDC, n.d. 3). Another useful resource for current evidence about both non-fatal and fatal fall rates is the CDC's Web-based Injury Statistics Query and Reporting System (WISQARS). This interactive database provides customized reports which are easily retrievable for various states in the nation (Figure 1).

TABLE 1. **National Ranking, Age-Groups, and Total Numbers of Deaths Due to Falls by Unintentional Injury, 1999–2010.**

Age-group	Rank	Total Number of Deaths
85+	1	512,415
75–84	1	584,521
65–74	1	571,349
55–64	1	881,178
45–54	1	925,945
35–44	1	723,904
25–34	1	781,424
15–24	2	882,214
10–14	2	600,403
5–9	1	682,972
1–4	1	928,693
<1	1	145,406

(Source: CDC, n.d. 1).

TABLE 2. **National Ranking and Age-Groups Affected by Unintentional Non-Fatal Injuries Due to Falls, 1999–2010.**

Age-group	Rank	Total Number of Non-Fatal Injuries
85+	1	512,415
75–84	1	584,521
65–74	1	571,349
55–64	1	881,178
45–54	1	925,945
35–44	1	723,904
25–34	1	781,424
15–24	2	882,214
10–14	2	600,403
5–9	1	682,972
1–4	1	928,693
<1	1	145,406

(Source: CDC, n.d. 1).

Levels of Prevention

Findings from the population-level data provided by the Centers for Disease Control and Prevention help us understand the importance of evidenced-based interventions for falls and injury prevention at the individual patient level. Falls and fall-related injury are public health problems of enormous concern not only because of their frequency within certain age-groups, but also because of their degree of preventability within these age-groups once identified. So, while age is important, knowing the types of exposures (risks) encountered and a fall's place of occurrence is even more useful, as nurses can focus evidenced-based interventions targeted to communities at the highest risk for fall injury and fall fatality. Public health is concerned with the health and wellbeing of the public, and as it relates to falls, providers typically focus their interventions using various levels of prevention.

As it relates to falls and injury prevention, a focus on risk factor reduction among known intrinsic and extrinsic risks is critical. Two useful public health frameworks for both falls reduction and injury prevention based on risk factor are the Haddon Matrix and the levels of prevention presented by Hugh Leavell (Katz, Wild, Elmore & Lucan, 2013). William Haddon's epidemiological injury framework recognizes three phases of injury prevention: pre-injury phase, injury phases and post-injury phase with respect to three potential causes of injury—human beings, vehicles and equipment, and the environment. Based on these factors of injury phases and potential causes, healthcare providers interact with patients to either minimize or eliminate risks altogether. For instance in the pre-injury phase, environmental assessment may reveal the presence of a throw rug on the landing of a staircase which could pose a tripping hazard to an elderly patient descending the steps. Removal of the rug eliminates that particular hazard altogether during the pre-injury phase.

Healthcare professionals focus care for the public around three levels of prevention. According to Leavell, level of prevention varies according to the presence or absence of risk factors and disease state (Katz, Wild, Elmore & Lucan, 2013). The three levels with application to public health prevention enforced by healthcare providers are primary, secondary and tertiary.

Primary Prevention

In the pre-disease state, goals center on primary prevention. In individuals who have no known risk factors for falls, primary prevention centers on health promotion activities. An example is a healthy 60-year-old residing in the community with no fall history who participates in Tai Chi to maintain his or her balance. Also in the pre-disease state are persons susceptible to the disease. An example is an osteoporotic female who is susceptible to bone fracture, but who has not yet suffered a fracture. Primary prevention focuses on specific protection through education and information such as ensuring adequate calcium, vitamin D, and exercise.

Secondary Prevention

Screening measures are often employed by healthcare professionals through history-taking and also through the use of falls risk assessment tools. These measures can detect the occurrence of a prior fall and also identify areas in which a person's risk can be reduced. In cases where the person is falling repeatedly, secondary prevention measures seek to reduce the possibility of future fall recurrence(s). This approach is more detailed than primary prevention measures and when the fall is a result of multiple factors, the analysis becomes more complex. Here the secondary prevention of additional falls will depend on correct identification of the exact risk factors and events responsible for the initial fall or falls. Obtaining a detailed fall-focused history, a focused physical examination, thorough environmental assessment, behavioral assessment and other types of assessments to try to pin-point why the fall occurred in the first place can help immensely in secondary prevention. Steps 1 through 3 of the five steps to falls prevention provide sufficient detail to answer the question of why the fall occurred, then allowing the nurse in Step 4 to formulate a working diagnosis of the various categories of falls which may have occurred.

Tertiary Prevention

Tertiary prevention is concerned with symptomatic disease care. Interventions center on reducing further disability and impairment. For individuals who fall frequently and incur serious injury such as hip fracture or head injury, the goals are to prevent further reductions in mobility and, if possible, to become rehabilitated without incurring further injury.

Where People Fall: Place of Occurrence

The Centers for Disease Control and Injury Prevention survey and tabulate not only age-groups affected by fatal and non-fatal fall injuries, but also common places of fall occurrence. Knowledge of the fall's place of occurrence helps nurses to streamline interventions for falls and injury prevention and serves as a useful benchmark for public policy officials who measure progress aggregately within databases.

People of all ages fall in both public and private settings such as in parking lots, off roof tops, from ladders in residential settings, in their homes, as well as in emergency departments, acute care hospitals, or in long term care settings. Some of the more classic fall scenarios, which have caught the attention of national organizations based on data-based evidence, are presented in Table 3. Among these examples include falls and fall-related injuries among children, ages 1–3, adults ages 18–64 and adults over 85 years of age.

Because fall-related injury deaths occur within certain age-groups, places, and certain exposures, nurses can target prevention screening efforts to prevent falls and fall-related injuries among those known to be at greatest risk.

Falls and Fall-related Injuries among Children

Falls are a leading cause of non-fatal injuries in all children. According to the CDC (see Table 3), about 8,000 children are treated in emergency departments for fall-related injuries, which adds up to almost 2.8 million children each year. Not only do these falls and injuries occur during sports, they occur in the home when children are unsupervised. Mechanisms for falls in the home include falling down steps and also out of windows during the spring and summer months. The CDC seeks to inform, educate and empower people to make a difference through prevention tips. (The CDC website is in Table 3).

Falls and Fall-related Injuries among Adults in the Workplace

According to the CDC's Morbidity and Mortality Weekly Report, occupational ladder fall injuries in 2011 in the United States accounted for 43% of all fatal falls (CDC, 2011; Table 3). Fall injury prevention research for strategies and solutions to prevent ladder falls are conducted through the National Institute for Occupational Safety and Health (NIOSH). Recent developments include the creation of apps for mobile devices which have a multimodal indicator and graphic orientation for ladder selection, inspection and positioning. (The CDC website is in Table 3).

Falls and Fall-related Injuries among Older Adults

Falls and fall-related injuries are highest among adults over age 65. For persons 65 and over, fatal and non-fatal fall-related injuries rank number one in the nation. Among older adults living in the community, nearly 1 of 3 falls each year, and for those in long-term care settings, nearly 50% of the 1.5 million residents incur falls (CDC, 2014). The CDC spotlights many publications and resources for preventing falls in the home, during recreation and in public places. (The CDC website is in Table 3).

Language and Terms Used to Describe Falls within Public Health

Within the public health domain, international and national organizations as well as professional societies charged with falls and injury prevention have developed standard terminology discussed below as well as signage about falls to help clarify what is meant by a fall event (American Hospital Association [AHA], American Geriatrics and British Geriatrics Society (AGS/ BGS) Task Force Clinical Practice Guidelines for Prevention of Falls in Oder Persons, National Quality Forum [NQF], The Joint Commission, the American Nurses Association [ANA], National Council on Aging [NCOA], Falls Free America, Prevention of Falls Network Europe [ProFane], Agency for Healthcare Research and Quality [AHRQ], Veteran's Administration National Center for Patient Safety [NCPS], Centers for Disease Control and Prevention [CDC], National Center for Injury Prevention and Control [NCIPC]).

From a population-based perspective, signage can facilitate a broad-based understanding of fall events occurring from environmental hazards, without spoken words. Common examples in the public domain include the use of yellow or red signs with a stick-figure of a patient who has tumbled to the ground. Placing these signs in the healthcare environment sends a non-verbal message acknowledging the importance of environmental safety and environmental hazards to patients, staff and visitors. Not only does signage provide a common sense approach to educating the public about falls occurring in the environment/patient care setting, but also use of simple language and icons on bed posters was found to reduce patient falls in one study (Dykes, Carroll & Hurley, 2010).

The science of falls and injury prevention is predicated on use of the best evidence gleaned from prior randomized and controlled fall prevention trials. Important work conducted through a systematic review by Cochrane shows a wide range of case definitions and methods are used to measure falls. Of some 90 publications, 44 provided no definition of the term fall (Hauer, Lamb, Jorstad, Todd & Becker, 2006). Public health reporting mechanisms within states and across federal agencies utilize various fall terminologies within administrative and public health surveillance systems to capture and collect data on fall events. Some of the more common terminology used by organizations responsive to falls prevention, providers observing falls and patients

TABLE 3. Classic Places, Causes, and Public Health Interventions for Falls among Various Ages.

Age-group	Place of Fall Occurrence	Scenarios and Type of Fall	Types of Public Health Interventions	CDC Web
1 to 3 years	Staircase in private home;	Child in rolling walker, not directly supervised incurs accidental fall	Educate and inform consumers: to use stair gates;	Protect the Ones You Love: Child Injuries are Preventable. Falls: The Reality. Available at: www.cdc.gov/safechild/Falls/index.html?source=govdelivery.
	From an open window	Child plays in room unsupervised with open window	Install guards on windows above ground level; window alarms	
18 to 64 years	Off a ladder in the workplace	Ladder is unsteady or unsecure, or worker missteps incurs accidental fall	Workforce training; enforcement of equipment safety in the environment (for instance, ladder safety devices/ alarms attached to ladder)	Fall Injuries Prevention in the Workplace. Available at: www.cdc.gov/niosh/topics/falls.
85+ years	Fall while descending the steps in one's home	Resident slips on throw rug placed on the landing surface of the steps	Home safety checks performed by nurses and/or consumers	Falls—Older Adults. Available at: www.cdc.gov/HomeandRecreationalSafety/Falls/Index.html.

Source: (CDC, 2011)

experiencing falls are discussed (Table 4). Note the various uses of the term "fall" and the importance of characteristics used to describe fall events by providers and patients.

TABLE 4. **Sample of Fall Definitions Used by Patients, Providers, and Organizations.**

National Organizational & Government Terminology [a]	Provider Terminology [b]	Patient Terminology [c]
Patient Fall	Fall(s)	"Suddenly went down…"
(Fall-related event)	Faller	"The bad one…"
Patient fall with injury	Frequent falls/ recurrent falls	"Serious fall…"
Sentinel event	Near fall	
	High risk to fall	
	Low risk to fall	
	No risk to fall	

Key= a/b. (National Quality Forum /American Nurses Association; Ambulatory Surgical Centers Quality Collaborative; Joint Commission on Accreditation; Prevention of Falls Network Europe); c. (Gray-Miceli, 2001).

Fall Terminology Used by National Organizations and within Public Health

As a variable, falls are monitored by many administrative and government surveillance systems. Within state government, for instance, the CDC has developed the telephone-administered health survey called the Behavioral Risk Factor Surveillance System (BRFSS). The BRFSS collects data about population health, including falls and falls with injury. Administrative officials from each state government administer the BRFSS questionnaire to a sample of residents within their state. BRFSS data is compiled and publically available through the Health Indicators Sortable Stats (CDC, n.d. 2). Part of the questionnaire includes core questions on falls and fall with injury and asks about fall frequency within the past three months. Falls are also sampled from community-dwelling populations when they come into contact with a healthcare organization or provider unit. In order for a healthcare agency to participate in Medicare reimbursement, the agency must collect the outcomes and assessment information set, or OASIS-C questionnaire (Centers for Medicare and Medicaid Services, OASIS-C, 2014). The OASIS inquires focus on the patient fall-risk assessment. In long-term care, the Minimum Data Set (MDS) 3.0 Quality Measures uses the term "fall within 180 days" as a trigger to guide further assessment of the resident (CMS, Medicare Quality, 2014). Because of the high prevalence of preventable injuries associated with patient falls, the current focus is falls with injury (NCPS, 2013; AHA, 2013).

Case Definitions of Falls by National Organizations

Patient Fall

Patient falls, or lack thereof, are a marker of quality of care by nurses. As a quality of care indicator within the healthcare setting, patient falls are defined by the National Quality Forum and the American Nurses Association as, "[A]n unplanned descent to the floor (or extension of the floor, e.g. trash can or other equipment) with or without injury. All types of falls are included, whether they result from physiological reasons or environmental reasons" (ANA, 2005).

Patient Fall with Injury

As nurses attempt to drive down the high rates of injurious fall in practice, it is important to recognize the relative value of determining the unit's fall injury rate so comparisons can be made within units over time and across similar types of facilities.

The American Nurses Association stipulates all documented patient falls with an injury level of minor or greater on eligible units in a calendar quarter are to be reported. These injuries should be reported as injury falls per 1000 Patient Days (National Quality Forum, 2014).

This formula for measuring falls with injury is:

(Total number of falls with injury ÷ Bed days of care) × 1,000

This same formula can be used to estimate specific levels of injury severity. For instance, to compute the number of falls with major injury, the numerator becomes total number of falls with major injury (defined a priori) divided by number of bed days of care × 1,000.

Sentinel Event

The Joint Commission refers to a fall event as a sentinel event when,

"[T]here is unexpected occurrence involving death or serious physical or psychological injury, or the risk thereof. Serious injury specifically includes loss of limb or function. The phrase "or the risk thereof" includes any process variation for which a recurrence would carry a significant chance of a serious adverse outcome."

Sentinel events signal the need for immediate investigation and response (TJC, 2011).

Provider Terminology

The range of terminology used by healthcare providers to describe patient falls in practice varies. Patient falls are typically viewed in the administrative data sets as dichotomous events requiring a yes or no response. Terminology used by healthcare researchers all reference the "faller", especially if the person falls more than once. Here one might read passages in the research literature such as, "elderly fallers in this cohort study experienced ..." Reference of the falling individual as "faller" is a way to refer to the data and should not be used out of this context, for example, when speaking to the falling person themselves, as this term tends to depersonalize a highly personal experience.

Frequent Falls

Frequent falls and *recurrent falls* are used interchangeably. It is important to note that the number of falls and time period used to describe the frequency of falls may vary within different healthcare settings. For instance, does falling three times in one year qualify as a *frequent fall* or is *frequent fall* best defined as two or more falls in one year? Facility protocol will typically define a recurrent fall. In any case, consistency in use of the terms is of critical importance.

Near-Falls

Near-falls are events in which the person catches him or herself and does not fall to the ground as in the case of a *true* fall. In one research study, near falls were found to be more frequent than true falls, often occurring before the true fall and are potentially useful in predicting overall fall risk (Maidan et al., 2014). Near falls also occur when staff members ease the patient to the ground or lower level.

Patient Terminology to Describe Their Fall

In prior work, we have found that older adults' descriptions of falls from personal experiences range from phrases such as "went down," "the bad one," or "went flying." As well, falls often evoke emotional responses such as fear, anger or frustration, and feelings of hopelessness and helplessness. Careful attention to the words and phrases used by a patient to describe their fall can help in further identification of the impact the fall has had in their life (Gray-Miceli, 2001).

Risk to Fall

Risk to fall has been further defined by outcomes obtained from use of fall risk assessment tools. Definitions of various degrees of risk (i.e. high, low or no risk to fall) vary across tools and in general outcomes from these tools have been used to streamline interventions. Careful attention should be paid to risk to fall and risk to injure, which are two very different types of assessments.

Risk to Fall and Risk to Injure: Use of Fall Risk Screening Tools

Current approaches to falls and injury prevention rest on a careful history of falls and injury risk examination of why the fall occurred. The examination is based on identifying potential factors that can be modified or treated and on primary prevention efforts to screen populations at risk for falls. While there are numerous published fall risk tools utilized with various patient populations, it should be noted that "no evidence-based instrument exists that can accurately identify older adult at risk for falling" (U.S. Preventive Services Task Force, 2012). The single most reliable risk factor to predict future falls in the elderly is a history of falling (AMDA, 2011). Therefore, typically the outcome of any fall risk assessment is the notation of an increased risk to fall or not, along with areas of deficits or impairments that research evidence substantiates. The outcome of a typical fall risk assessment should be the identification of modifiable fall risk factors.

Since fall risk assessment tools provide a temporary indication of patient risk, care must be taken in the interpretation of the findings. Nurses must always go with their best judgment about a patient's safety risk. For instance, just because fall risk assessment tool findings indicate that the patient is *not at risk to fall*, this does not always mean that they won't fall. The reason for this is two-fold. Firstly, baseline physiology changes; so, for example, while a patient may have a normal physiological blood pressure at 10 am when the fall risk screen is performed, at 10:05 they could have an acute perforation of their bowel, become hypotensive, and fall. The second reason is that the content included on fall risk screening assessment tools does not capture the multitude of events and pathology implicated in all falls which occur for different reasons. Of note, there are different types of patient falls and fall risk tools used in hospitals that are only for anticipated physiological falls (for instance those due to acute or chronic conditions).

As a screening measure for persons who have not fallen, upon admission, and with any change in the level of care, community agencies as well as acute and long-term care facilities require nurses to perform a falls risk assessment.

Used prior to any fall occurrence, the falls risk assessment tool helps to identify where to pinpoint additional assessment and intervention. Typically facilities will have individual fall risk protocol and direct the nurse as to which assessment tool is required. As part of the health history of the fall, a falls risk assessment is performed to screen for the history of falling and also as part of the post-fall analysis. Assessments of risk to fall are delivered by healthcare professionals and trained non-professionals. For older adult populations, the fall risk assessment is a diagnostic process intended to determine an older person's risk of falling in order to plan coordinated treatment and long-term follow-up. The assessment includes methods that are specifically designed and tested for the measurement of risk of falling, e.g., gait speed, static balance, strength, cardiovascular assessment (Lamb, Jørstad-Stein, Hauer, & Becker, 2005).

Using a population approach perspective, age group, type of living environment, and condition of the patient, (e.g., behavior, presence of impairment, disease and medication use) place a person at risk to fall. As science evolves, we continue to learn more about risks to fall. When delivering care to any patient, nurses must be knowledgeable about fall risks. Nurses can stay informed by accessing the latest evidence relative to patient risk factors to fall. Nurses often refer to current Clinical Practice Guidelines (CPGs) in out-patient ambulatory settings and for current recommendations from professional societies for falls and injury prevention. How risk factors, whether in isolation or combination, contribute to fall risk will vary among patient populations and age-groups. Recommendations for interventions based on these risk factors are housed on web-based platforms, but some of the more commonly used web-based resources are presented at the end of this chapter.

Assessment for falls risk involves many of the parameters listed in Table 5, among other factors. These parameters may exist as permanent or temporary. Risk factors within an individual have been referred to as intrinsic factors, whereas those as a result of a situation or context external to the individual are referred to as extrinsic. Evidence from Chang's seminal work drawn from a meta-analysis of randomized clinical trials, shows older adult falls are typically due to multiple risks and also, that interventions for the prevention of falls are best if they involve a multidisciplinary component.

Modifiable or Potentially Reversible Fall Risk Factors

Among the known intrinsic and extrinsic risks to fall are risk factors that are considered by experts to be modifiable. 'Modifiable' means there is a potential for reversibility. If these modifiable factors are detected early in

TABLE 5. Common Iintrinsic and Extrinsic Risk Factors to Fall and Examples of How These Factors Increase Risk to Fall.

Intrinsic Risk Factor	Category	Example of how the factor and category increase risk to fall
Sensory dysfunction	Visual impairment	Patient has limited ability or inability to view their environment.
	Peripheral neuropathy	Patient can not feel their feet on the floor, posing difficulty with foot placement and walking.
Gait impairment	Ataxic gait	Patient's gait is unsteady, erratic or wobbly with ambulation.
Balance impairment	Loss of balance due to muscle weakness	Patient experiences difficulty or inability to maintain upright posture either sitting or standing and experiences loss of balance.
	Loss of balance post-stroke	Patient experiences difficulty or inability to maintain upright posture either sitting or standing and experiences loss of balance.
Alteration in level of consciousness/ mental status	Post-operative sedation	Patient has difficulty sustaining attention or is unable to do so; patient loses concentration or focus on the task at hand.
	Use of anesthesia	Patient has difficulty sustaining attention or is unable to do so; patient loses concentration or focus on the task at hand.
	Delirium	Patient's level of consciousness waxes and wanes along with loss of concentration or focus on the task at hand.
Physiological changes in vital signs	Orthostatic hypotension	Patient's blood pressure drops significantly with standing or sitting up, potentially resulting in loss of balance.
Urinary dysfunction	Urge urinary incontinence	Patient has a urinary accident on the floor and slips, or patient has urgency to urinate and hurries to the bathroom where a slip or loss of footing occurs.
Psychological	Depression	
Generalized weakness/debility	Sarcopenia; muscle weakness/wasting	Patient experiences loss of strength or diminished leg strength, making standing upright difficult without assistance.
Patient footwear	Inappropriate footwear (socks; barefoot)	Patient has difficulty with ambulation due to poorly fitting shoes, use of high heels, slippery socks, or absence of footwear entirely; contact with floor surface area then causes a slip or fall.
Extrinsic Risk Factor	Category	Example of how it the factor and category increase risk to fall.
	Use of assistive device	Patient has difficulty using the ambulation equipment and may walk into objects or persons; patient cannot recall how to use the device; the device itself is unsteady or has poor contact surface areas causing slipping when in contact with surface area.
	Frayed carpeting	Patients shoe or heel gets caught in frayed carpet causing a fall.
High Risk Medications/ETOH use	Any medication that has a side effect of drowsiness or sedation	Side effects of the medication alter the patient's ability to sustain attention or concentrate; patient may become confused.
Risky Behavior	Climbing an unsteady ladder with no contact guarding or arm rails	Climbing unsafely causes a loss of balance and a subsequent fall.

the pre-injury phase, then falls and fall-related injuries may potentially be avoided. Within the acute care setting (Oliver, Healy & Haines, 2010) has identified several modifiable risk factors in the list below. The means of fall injury reduction and falls prevention are the early identification of these factors and the monitoring of the health status of the patient. Note that not all fall risk assessment tools use these methods. So, rather than thinking about patients as high or low risk, all patients should be considered at risk to fall and evaluated for these modifiable risk factors.

Factors considered modifiable and capable of averting patient falls and fall-related injuries:

- High-risk medications (sedatives/hypnotics/anti-anxiety agents)
- Alcohol intoxication
- Delirium
- Behavioral agitation
- Syncope
- Urinary frequency and incontinence
- Visual impairment
- Gait and balance disturbances
- Profound weakness, fatigue
- Unstable vital signs
- Orthostatic hypotension
- Laboratory abnormalities: Low platelet count, anemia, sepsis, hypoglycemia, hyperglycemia

It is important to note that there are many case examples where patients have been deemed at no risk to fall using a falls risk assessment tool, and they actually do fall, for reasons not captured by the risk assessment tool. A classic example is a fall due to acute events and anticipated physiologic falls. Consider the following case of Mrs. P.

Case example of a patient admitted to the sub-acute unit of a long-term care facility for management of acute lymphocytic leukemia (ALL)

Following her second bout of ALL, Mrs. P and her physician decided her care could best be managed in an outpatient setting such as a sub-acute unit. The plan included daily administration of fresh frozen platelets in a supervised sub-acute unit of a nearby nursing home. Mrs. P, a 70-year-old female, drove to the nursing home for treatment which was anticipated to last 7–10 days. Upon admission to the unit, Mrs. P received a falls risk assessment by the intake registered nurse. A standard tool was used, and it indicated that she had no risks to fall. Questions on the falls risk assessment asked about prior fall history for which she scored none or zero (0); history of more than three chronic illnesses, for which she had only one, thus she was scored at zero (0); use of high risk medications, such as sedatives, hypnotics and anti-anxiety agents, for which she had none, score (0); and other classic questions about visual, gait and balance impairment for which she scored zero (0). In sum, her fall risk score indicated she had no risks to fall. On review of systems during the initial history however, it was noted that Mrs. P was extremely fatigued and had felt generalized weakness for the past month.

Although a plan of care based on no risks to fall may have been appropriate based on the assessment tool results, the nurse still lowered the height of the bed, raised bed rails at night, kept a night light on, and made frequent clinical rounds every morning to check on Mrs. P.

Since Mrs. P was ambulatory, independent in all activities of daily living, the nurse thought to allow Mrs. P to walk to the bathroom to use the toilet. In fact, the physician's orders gave no indication that she would need assistance at all. Orders read "up ad lib." On the second day of admission, the patient began to receive fresh frozen platelets and white blood cells via transfusion. She also had her hemoglobin and platelets checked every six hours on the first, second and third day of admission. Her baseline hemoglobin was 7.2 with a hematocrit of 26. An absolute platelet count was read at <30.

On the evening of the second night, Mrs. P lowered the side rail, got up from bed and walked to the bathroom to urinate. While in the bathroom she lost her footing when turning and fell hitting her head on the sink. She was dazed but managed to get back into bed independently. Two hours later when the nurse came to her bedside to administer the platelets, she noticed a large laceration over her eyebrow which was oozing serous material. Remembering that Mrs. P had no falls risk, she told her to call when she had to get up again and left the room to get a bandage. The nurse became busy due to low staffing and never returned to check on her. Mrs. P was pronounced dead the following morning when she was found by the morning staff. Family caregivers, administration, the physician and staff were shocked and all questioned what happened.

Questions to consider: Was this patient truly at no risk to fall even though the fall risk tool indicated no risk to fall? Did the nurse exercise correct judgment in allowing Mrs. P to ambulate to the toilet independently given her complaints of fatigue and weakness and laboratory evidence of anemia and low platelet count? What could the nurse have done once she discovered the head injury?

With hindsight it is easy to see what went wrong. The nurse's judgment about the patient condition in terms of risk for injury from a potential fall and the need to promote the safety of the patient such as through safe mobility were missing. Mrs. P was indeed at high risk to fall and injury due to an acute underlying disease and other physiological reasons. Placing the patient on routine observation, and frequent vital sign checks from the day of admission as well as providing assistance to the toilet or using a bed pan would have likely averted this fall. Once Mrs. P fell and hit her head, she should have been placed on neurological checks every 15 minutes × 4 while the physician was notified. Transfer to the emergency room for diagnostic imaging of her head and monitoring for head injury would have been appropriate.

Fall Injury Reduction

While the current state of the science is replete with identification of risks to fall and underlying reasons responsible for a fall, our greatest concern as healthcare providers is to protect patients from harm and injury. Unintentional injuries due to falls are the leading causes of fatality in America across many age-groups, especially older Americans (CDC, NCIPC, 2014). In 2010, the National Center for Health Statistics reported injuries due to falls were the most common condition prevalent in the emergency room by elderly nursing home residents and were potentially preventable (NCHS, 2010). In the hospital setting, injuries due to falls are estimated to range from 30 to 51% (Oliver, Healy, & Haines, 2010) and are still noted to be the top adverse event in the acute care setting (Spoelstra, Given & Given, 2012).

Fall-related injuries are also significant in long-term care. In their seminal work on fall-related injuries, more than 2,400 admissions to the Veterans Administration Hospitals during a three year period were associated with 50% of patients incurring hip fracture and 10% with intracranial injuries, costing an average US $23,723 per admission. In non-Veterans' administration hospitals, rates of injuries were higher and the average cost was US $31,507 per admission (Quigley et al., 2012). Overall the cost burden (direct medical costs) of falls is estimated at $30 billion (Stevens, Corso, Finkelstein & Miller, 2006). There is an urgent need for interdisciplinary collaboration to develop and spread adoption of effective strategies for fall injury risk assessment and prevention/protection programs (Wyman, 2012).

Injury Severity

The National Center for Patient Safety has created a broad classification scheme for identifying types of injuries according to severity (NCPS, 2009). As seen in Table 6, both minor and major types of injuries occur, the most severe being a fatal fall injury resulting in death. Injury severity levels are also reported by the National Quality Forum and National Database of Nursing Quality indicators.

TABLE 6. Injury Severity by National Center for Patient Safety (2009).

Level	Type	Example
1	Minor injury	Abrasion, bruise, minor laceration; injuries that do not require substantial medical intervention and do not extend the patient's or resident's length of stay except for observation or test results.
2	Major injury	Hip fracture, head trauma, arm fracture; injuries that require substantial medical or surgical intervention, increase a patient's or resident's length of stay, or result in disfigurement or permanent loss of function with or without surgical repair.
3	Fatal fall injury	Death resulting from fall-related injuries not treatable by medical assistance.

Preventing Injurious Falls

Fall-related injuries can be devastating to the individual who falls. Ranging from minor to major injuries, it is the major injuries targeted for immediate reduction. To accomplish this requires an evidence base along with prudent practices that foster interprofessional collaboration and consistently involve the patient. Benefit and risks must also be included in the equation of deciding what is in a particular patient's best interest.

A population-based approach which identifies patients at greatest risk to injury has evolved that is embraced by the ABCS criteria discussed below (Boushon et.al., 2008). In addition to this, studies in long-term care facilities are finding that risks of incurring head injury are due to mobility status. In one analysis, ambulatory elderly residents living in an assisted living unit were more likely to incur head injures than those residing in a skilled nursing unit (Gray-Miceli, Ratcliffe & Thomasson, 2013).

A stands for "age" or evidence of physical frailty. Advanced age (over age 85), has been associated statistically with higher incidences of certain types of injurious falls. For instance, evidence collected by the National Center for Injury Prevention and Control (NCIPC) and the CDC show that fatal falls, traumatic brain injuries (TBIs), and hip fractures are highest among those 85 and older. Classic markers of physical frailty include decreased body mass index and reduced endurance and physical strength.

B stands for "bones" and patients with osteoporosis or prior hip fracture are at greatest risk. Other bone conditions where there is a loss of bone mass, such as rickets, seen in children, are also associated with a higher incidence of fracture injuries (CDC, 2014). Certain medications, such as chronic steroids, can result in loss of calcium from the bone and in osteoporosis. With advancing age, osteopenia occurs, often a prelude to osteoporosis. It has been estimated that more than 4.5 million women over age 50 suffer from osteoporosis (CDC, n.d. 5). Detection of osteoporosis is a critical primary prevention effort to reduce the incidence of preventable fractures. Additionally, cancer is a disease which can metastasize to the bone. Careful follow-up for bone lyses due to cancer is critical in an effort to reduce injuries associated with impact from a fall.

C stands for "coagulation disorder" related to anti-coagulation. Anti-coagulation states are sought repeatedly and therapeutically, such as in the case of a patient with a history of blood clots. Conditions such as immobility following a hip fracture repair places a patient at increased risk for blood clots or deep vein thrombosis, and therefore medications are used to minimize this risk. In addition to medication, certain diseases are associated with anti-coagulation states; placing the patient at higher risk for injury associated with blood loss should a fall occur. One common condition, thrombocytopenia, produces a significant drop in the absolute number of platelets, a clotting ingredient in normal blood. Other conditions arise from use of medications such as Warfarin or Coumadin. Certain anti-platelet medications were found to be associated with increased risk for mortality from a head injury (Ohm, Mina, Howells, Bair, Bendick, 2005).

S stands for "surgery"; specifically, recent surgery. Patients who have undergone recent surgery have an incision, which causes pain and an alteration in muscle, tissue, and bone or skin integrity. These conditions cause patients temporary physical impairment, thus increasing their risk for additional injury. Post-operative pain is a potent distracter in daily living, also referred to as the fifth vital sign.

Measuring Falls

In a prior study only 41% used prospective data collection methods with the vast majority relying on past recall or retrospective analysis (Hauer, Lamb, Jorstad, Todd & Becker, 2006). Measuring falls using past fall recall and retrospective analysis is very problematic for several reasons. The true prevalence of falls for the population will likely be inaccurate, as falls might be omitted from the count if they are unobserved, unreported, or not witnessed by patients or staff. This does little in the overall analysis nurse's need to make for individual patients when determining their fall frequency and overall plan of care for reduction. One of the best methods for measurement of falls is prospective continuous monitoring. Nurse managers typically accomplish this through analysis of their 30-day monthly reports wherein falls are aggregated among patient populations. Computerized programs are also commercially available to trend fall data electronically and to signal staff when patient falls exceed the individual baseline.

Mechanisms for Patient Falls within Healthcare Facilities

Creating and maintaining an organizational culture of safety for excellence in quality of care and patient safety has potential to eliminate falls altogether. A sample of factors identified by the post-fall analysis within a healthcare facility is provided in Table 7. Over a nine-year period, 2002–2013, multiple root causes for falls within an acute care hospital were noted, spanning leadership, assessment issues, care planning, and patient education.

Types of Patient Falls

When thinking about falls and injury prevention, the nurse provider must recognize falls occur from very specific etiological factors subsumed within broader categories such as human factors. How providers think about fall classification likely influence subsequent preventive action. For example, if one believes or determines a patient fall is solely due to an accident, then one is likely to recommend patient's to "accident-proof" their home. So too, falls due to acute physiological events are managed differently by healthcare providers than falls due to environmental accidents. For these reasons, a few researchers have classified sub-types of falls according to various underlying phenomena implicated through empiric findings in the fall. Based on these two prior empiric studies in either acute care hospitals (Morse, 1997) or long-term care/nursing home settings (Gray-Miceli, 2010) two distinct classification schemes for falls have been developed by nurse researchers who analyzed

TABLE 7. **Root Cause Information for Fall-Related Events Reviewed by The Joint Commission from 2004 to June 2013.**

Root Cause of Fall-related Event	Frequency of occurrences
Assessment	436
Leadership	335
Communication	329
Human factors	323
Physical environment	219
Care planning	125
Information management	77
Continuum of care	48
Special interventions	42
Patient education	41

Source: The Joint Commission, 2011.

and cataloged the various types of patient falls and their likely responsible underlying mechanism (Table 8). Additional detail about terminology used by Morse and/or Gray-Miceli in their classification scheme can be found from the original seminal research.

The standard of care calls for mandatory components of health history and physical examination which must be asked and completed among all populations if falls and fall related injuries are to be prevented. Therefore, clinical decisions made to determine that a fall was likely due to an accident or due to an acute underlying medical event must be reflected in the fall-focused patient history, physical examination and environmental assessment as detailed in the first three steps of *Five Easy Steps to Prevent Falls*. Falls with injury can occur within any of these broad classifications included in Table 8.

Organization of This Book

The contents of *Five Easy Steps to Prevent Falls* are in five succinct chapters. Each step relates directly to one or more of the Ten Essential Public Health Services (PHS) broad objectives and brings the nurse and interprofessional team closer to reducing falls and fall-related injuries within the United States. Note that use of the term *community* in the context of this book refers broadly to patient care settings where nurses encounter patients at risk to fall or those who have already fallen in a location such as the home, an acute care setting or a long-term care setting. *Community* also broadly includes other

TABLE 8. **Sample of Terminology Used for Fall Classifications by Nurse Researchers.**

Morse Classification of Patient Falls [a]	Gray-Miceli Classification of Patient Falls [b]
► Accidental fall	► Environment
► Anticipated	► Acute Medical
► Physiological fall	► Chronic Disease
	► Medication related
► Unanticipated	► Poor Safety Awareness
► Physiological fall	► Poor Judgment
	► Behavioral
	► Unknown

Key = a (Morse, 1997); b (Gray-Miceli et al., 2010).

team members working together to ensure patient safety and reduce falls and fall-related injuries. *Five Easy Steps to Prevent Falls* is organized as follows:

Step 1: Eliciting a Fall-Focused Health History

Broad PHS Objective: Monitoring the health status to identify and solve community problems

Step 2: Conducting a Fall-Focused Physical Assessment

Broad PHS Objective: Monitoring the health status to identify and solve community problems

Step 3: Detecting Environmental Hazards & Modifying the Environment for Patient and Healthcare Worker Safety

Broad PHS Objective: Diagnosing and investigating health problems and health in the community

Broad PHS Objective: Assuring a competent workforce

Step 4: Diagnosing the Fall Type and Developing an Interprofessional Team Plan of Care

Broad PHS Objective: Diagnosing and investigating health problems and health in the community

Broad PHS Objective: Mobilizing community partnerships

Broad PHS Objective: Developing policies and plans that support individual and community health

Step 5: Informing, Educating and Empowering Patients

Broad PHS Objective: Inform, educate and empower people

References

Agency for Healthcare Research and Quality (AHRQ). *National Guideline Clearinghouse. Guideline Summary NGC-9721. Fall Prevention.*

American Geriatrics Society and British Geriatrics Society Panel on Prevention of Falls in Older Persons. (2011). Summary of the updated American Geriatrics Society/ British Geriatrics Society clinical practice guideline for prevention of falls in older persons. *Journal of the American Geriatrics Society, 59*, 148–157.

American Medical Directors Association. (AMDA). (2011). Falls and fall risk. In *Clinical Practice Guidelines in the LTC setting.*

American Nurses Association. (2005). National Database for Nursing Quality Indicators®. Guidelines for data collection and submission on quarterly indicators, version 5.0

American Nurses Association. (2012). *Principles for nurse staffing* (2nd ed.). Silver Spring, MD: Author.

American Nurses Association. (2013). *Safe patient handling and mobility: Interprofessional national standards.* Silver Spring, MD: Author.

Boushon, B., Nielson, G., Quigley, P., Rutherford, P., Taylor, J., & Shannon, D. (2008). *Transforming care at the bedside how-to-guide: Reducing patient injuries from falls.* Cambridge, MA: Institute for Healthcare Improvement. Retrieved from http://www.ihi.org/resources/Pages/Tools/TCABHowToGuideReducing PatientInjuriesfromFalls.aspx

Centers for Disease Control and Prevention (CDC). (2011). *Surveillance for traumatic brain injury related deaths in the U.S. 1997–2007.* MMWR Surveillance Summaries 60:5. Rockville, MD: Author

Centers for Disease Control and Prevention (CDC). (2014). *The public health system and the 10 essential public health services.* Retrieved from http://www.cdc.gov/nphpsp/essentialservices.html

Centers for Disease Control and Injury Prevention and Control (CDC). (n.d. 1) Retrieved from www.webapp.cdc.gov/cgi-bin/broker.exe?_Program=wisqnf.nfile

Centers for Disease Control and Prevention (CDC). (n.d. 2). *Sortable risk factors and health indicators* [Data set]. Retrieved from http://wwwn.cdc.gov/sortablestats/

Centers for Disease Control and Prevention. (CDC). (n.d. 3) *Unintentional fatal fall injuries in nursing homes.* Retrieved from http:www.cdc.gov/injury/wisqars

Centers for Disease Control and Prevention. (CDC). (n.d. 4). *Falls among older adults: An overview.* Retrieved from http://www.cdc.gov/homeandrecreationalsafety/falls/adultfalls.html

Centers for Disease Control and Prevention. (CDC). (n. d. 5). *Osteoporosis.* Retrieved from http://www.cdc.gov/nchs/fastats/osteoporosis.htm

Chang, J. T., Morton, S. C., Rubenstein, L. Z., ... Shekelle, P. G. (2004). Interventions for the prevention of falls in older adults: Systematic review and meta-analysis of randomized clinical trials. *British Medical Journal, 328*, 680.

Dykes, P. C., Carroll, D. L., & Hurley, A., (2010). Fall prevention in acute care hospitals: a randomized trial. *Journal of the American Medical Association, 304*, 1912–1918.

Gray-Miceli, D. (2001). *A phenomenological study of the meaning of serious falls to older adults.* Doctoral diss., Widener University.

Gray-Miceli, D., Ratcliffe, S. J. & Thomasson, A. (2013). Ambulatory assisted living elderly fallers at greatest risk for head injury. *Journal of the American Geriatrics Society, 61*, 1817–1819. doi: 10.1111/jgs.12467

Hauer, K., Lamb, S. E., Jorstad, E. C., Todd, C., & Becker, C. (2006). Systematic review of definitions and methods of measuring falls in randomised controlled fall prevention trials. *Age and Aging, 35*, 5–10.

Institute of Medicine. (1988). *The future of public health.* Washington, DC:

National Academies Press. Retrieved from http://books.nap.edu/openbook. php?record_id=1091

The Joint Commission. (2011). *Comprehensive accreditation manual for behavioral health care: Refresher course,* January. Available at http:www.JCAHO

Katz, D. L., Wild, D., Elmore, J. G., & Lucan, S. C. (2013). *Jekel's epidemiology, biostatistics, preventive medicine, and public health.* St. Louis: Elsevier Health Sciences.

Kansas Department of Aging, Workgroup 05. Incident Report Form.

Lamb, S. E., Jørstad-Stein, E. C., Hauer, K., & Becker, C. (2005). Development of a common outcome data set for fall injury prevention trials: the Prevention of Falls Network Europe consensus. *Journal of the American Geriatric Society, 53,* 1618–1622.

Maidan, I., Freedman, T., Tzemah, R., Giladi, N., Mirelman, A., & Hausdorff, J. M. (2014). Introducing a new definition of a near fall: intra-rater and inter-rater reliability. *Gait Posture, 39,* 645–647.

Morse, J. 1997. *Preventing patient falls.* Thousand Oaks, CA: Sage.

National Center for Patient Safety (NCPS). (2013). *Falls toolkit.* Retrieved from http://www.patientsafety.va.gov/professionals/onthejob/falls.asp

National Council on Aging (NCOA). (2005). *Falls free: Promoting a national falls prevention action plan.* Washington, DC: Author. Retrieved from http://www.ncoa.org/improve-health/center-for-healthy-aging/content-library/FallsFree_NationalActionPlan_Final.pdf

Ohm C., Mina, A., Howells, G., Bair, H., & Bendick, P. (2005). Effects of anti-platelet agents on outcomes for elderly patients with traumatic intracranial hemorrhage. *Journal of Trauma, 58,* 518–522.

Oliver, D., Healey, F., & Haines, T. (2010). Preventing falls and fall-related injuries in hospitals. *Clinical Geriatric Medicine, 26,* 645–692.

Quigley, P., Campbell, R. R., Bulat, T., Olney, R. L., Buerhaus, P., & Needleman, J. (2012).

Incidence and cost of serious fall-related injuries in nursing homes. *Clinical Nursing Research, 21,* 10–23.

Spoelstra, S. L., Given, B. A., & Given, C. W. (2012). Fall prevention in hospitals: An integrative review. *Clinical Nursing Research, 21,* 92–112

Stevens, J. A., Corso, P. S., Finkelstein, E. A., & Miller, T. R. (2006). The costs of fatal and non-fatal falls among older adults. *Injury Prevention, 12,* 290–295.

U.S. Preventive Services Task Force. (2012, May). *Prevention of falls in community-dwelling older adults.* Retrieved from http://www.uspreventiveservicestaskforce.org/uspstf/uspsfalls.htm

Wyman J. (2012). Commentary on incidence and cost of serious fall-related injuries in nursing homes. *Clinical Nursing Research, 21,* 6–9.

Useful web-based resources

American Geriatrics Society, British Geriatrics Society. (2010). AGS/BGS Clinical Practice Guidelines: *Prevention of falls in older persons.* New York: American Geriatrics Society. www.americangeriatrics.org/health_care_professionals/clinical_practice/clinical_guidelines_recommendations/2010.

American Nurses Association (ANA) workplace safety and patient safety resources: http://www.nursingworld.org/MainMenuCategories/WorkplaceSafety/Healthy-Work-Environment/SafePatient

BRFSS (The Behavioral Risk Factor Surveillance System) Health Indicators Sortable Stats; http://wwwn.cdc.gov/sortablestats/

Centers for Disease Control and Prevention, various falls prevention links:

www.cdc.gov/safechild/Falls/index.html?source=govdelivery

cdc.gov/HomeandRecreationalSafety/Falls/Index.html

cdc.gov/safechild/Falls/index.html?source=govdelivery

cdc.gov/niosh/topics/falls

Centers for Medicare and Medicaid Services, Partnership for Patients: partnershipforpatients.cms.gov b

Hartford Institute for Geriatric Nursing Consult Geri RN, a robust source of evidence-based and authoritative information about nursing care of older adults: http://consultgerirn.org/

Hughes R.G. (ed.). (2008). *Patient safety and quality: An evidence-based handbook for nurses.* (Prepared with support from the Robert Wood Johnson Foundation). AHRQ Publication No. 08-0043. Rockville, MD: Agency for Healthcare Research and Quality. Available at http://www.ahrq.gov/professionals/clinicians-providers/resources/nursing/resources/nurseshdbk/FrontMatter_NursesHandbook.pdf

International Classification of Diseases (ICD). http://www.who.int/classifications/icd/en/

The Joint Commission Sentinel Event Statistics: www.joint.commission.org/sentinel_event.aspx

National Council on Aging. www.ncoa.org/

National Center for Injury Prevention and Control (NCIPC): www.ncipc.gov/

National Quality Forum (NQF): www.quality.forum.org

Prevention of Falls Network Europe (ProFane). www.profane.eu.org

U.S. Preventive Task Force. Prevention of Falls in Community-Dwelling Older Adults: http://www.uspreventiveservicestaskforce.org/uspstf/uspsfalls.htm

Step 1. Eliciting a Fall-Focused Health History

Overview

The purpose of this chapter is to discuss the fall-focused health history obtained by the professional nurse during the medical encounter with the patient with a focus on those at greatest risk to fall and injure or those who have already fallen. For those who have already fallen, the history gathered is similar to other illness evaluations, and is focused on specific events leading to and occurring with the fall. The history must be as complete as possible, as it forms the basis of the overall plan of care for either reducing modifiable fall risks and/or preventing future falls and injury.

This chapter discusses obtaining information from the patient, family member, or caregiver in the fall-focused history. Content is organized around the major types of falls, as well as important leading questions to include when appropriate. Because falls and injury have the potential to affect all age groups, information is gathered for the groups listed below.

1. Patients who have never fallen, but who are susceptible and at risk due to presence of intrinsic or extrinsic fall risk factors;
2. Patients who have recently fallen (post-fall assessment and analysis); and
3. Patients at greater risk for fall-related injuries and modifiable falls, but not necessarily from a high-risk age group or population.

In addition, while completing all of the required elements of a fall-focused history, the information provided frames only half of the story: the healthcare provider's perspective. The other half of the story, which is of equal importance, is the patient's perspective, as well as that of family, caregivers, and anyone witness to the fall.

As part of the national recommendations for falls prevention in older adults over age 65 living in the community, a ten-step algorithm is available for healthcare professionals to follow (American Geriatrics Society, Falls Prevention, 2011). It begins with the fall history over the past one year. Depending on the patient response, the provider is directed to additional steps to assess. This algorithm is based on the latest compilation of the highest graded evidence concerning community-dwelling older adults. For additional information see or see www.medcats.com/FALLS/frameset.htm.

Broad Public Health Service Objective

Monitor health status to identify and solve community problems.

Educational Learner Outcomes

At the conclusion of this chapter, the learner should be able to:

1. Recognize the situational context (time, approach, baseline information, and special considerations) for gathering a complete fall-focused health history;
2. Incorporate historical medical information into the health history of the patient at-risk for falling;
3. Incorporate historical medical information into the health history of the patient at-risk for serious injury; and
4. Incorporate historical medical information into the health history of the patient who has fallen.

Learner Outcome 1: Recognizing the Situational Context

Recognize the situational context (baseline information, time, approach, and special considerations) for gathering a complete fall focused health history.

Before the Interview: Obtaining Baseline Health Information

Prior to interviewing the patient, the nurse will need to review the medical record to become familiar with the patient's medical history, risks to fall and injure, and/or information about his or her most recent fall. Having an existing trusting relationship with the patient or the ability to engender trust with the patient will help in obtaining the overall health history accurately as well as in implementing the post-fall plan of care. Typically, healthcare facility protocol requires an incident report to be completed upon admission to the facility. Most often the incident report is not specific to a fall event, but *any* incident such as loss of personal property or an altercation with an employee. The lack of focus on the fall event creates a situation where important medical or situational information about a fall is not included on the incident report. The Office of the Inspector General has noted in their seminal work issues related to patient harm when a hospital incident reporting system fails to capture necessary information (Department of Health and Human Services,

2012). In contrast, the Kansas Department of Aging's Working Group 5 has developed a standard incident report form to be used by administrative officials when gathering data about a fall or injury (see Figure 1-1). Note this incident report houses much more detail than the standard incident report used by facilities. Failure to capture the correct medical information surrounding the fall, in a timely manner (i.e., at the time of the fall), can create a delay in care. The Institute of Medicine addresses the issue of time-liness in its overarching framework for patient safety. Among others, patient care must be safe, equitable, efficient, and timely (see www.aha.org/advocacy-issues/quality/background.shtml).

FALL INCIDENT REPORT

(This tool is only an example. Please adapt it to meet the needs of your facility and residents.)

MR # _____ Last Name _____ First Name _____ Room # _____

Date _____ Time _____ am/pm □ Resident □ Employee □ Visitor

Type   of   Incident   (Check):   □   Fall   □   Behavior   □   Other (Specify):

_____

Physical Assessment:
If fall what position was person found in? (Describe in detail): _____

_____

Describe mobility or range-of-motion of extremities following incident: _____

_____

Is assessed mobility or range-of-motion ability a change? (Check): □ No □ Yes (Describe): _____

Injury (Check): □ None □ Laceration □ Skin Tear □ Abrasion □ Hematoma □ Swelling □ Other (Describe and Locate on Diagram): _____

Vital Signs: Other: B/P Lie _____ Temp _____ BG Accu Check _____

B/P Sit _____ Pulse _____ Pulse Oximetry _____

B/P Stand ___ Resp _____ Neuro Checks _____

Treatment (Check All That Apply)

□ Examined at Hospital: _____   □ Admitted to Hospital: _____

□ Xray Done (Results): _____   □ First Aid Administered: _____

_____

Name of Person(s) Administering Treatment: _____

Physician Notified: _____ Time: _____ am/pm **Response Time:** _____ am\pm

Family/Other Notified: _____ Time: _____ am/pm **Response Time:** _____ am/pm

(Complete Reverse at the Time of Incident)

Figure 1-1. Kansas Department of Aging Workgroup 05 Fall Incident Report Form (page 1 of 2).

Investigation

Exact Location of Incident (Check): □ Resident's Room □ Hallway □ Bathroom □ Nursing Station
□ Lobby □ Shower Room □ Dining Room □ Other (Specify room ##: hallway, bathroom, shower etc.)
□ Incident Witnessed **Name of Witness:** _____

Address of Witness: _____
□ Incident Un-Witnessed **Name of Person Who Discovered Incident:** _____

Description of Incident: _____
_____

Person(s) Involved, Statements About Incident: _____
_____
_____

What Was the Involved Person Attempting To Do: □ Getting Out of Bed □ Standing Still
□ Wheeling in W/C □ Walking □ Reaching for Object □ Transferring To/From Chair or W/C □ Going to the
Bathroom □ Need for Dry Incontinent □ Other (Specify): _____

Equipment Involved: □ Walker □ Cane/Crutch □ Wheelchair □ W/C Wheels Locked
□ W/C/Wheels Unlocked □ Geri-Chair □ G/C Back Reclined □ G/C Back Upright □ G/C Wheels Locked □ G/C
Wheels Unlocked □ Bed □ Half Bedrails □ Full Bedrails □ Bedrails Up □ Bedrails Down
□ No Bedrails □ Other (Specify): _____

Environment: □ Wet Floor □ Wet Floor Sign in Place □ No Sign □ Object on Walkway
□ Poor Lighting □ Rug in Walkway □ Clutter in Walkway □ Foot Ware (Specify) _____
□ New Admit □ Recent Room Move □ Call Light in Reach □ Call Light Not in Reach
□ Bed/Chair Alarm On □ Bed/Chair Alarm Off

Diagnosis or Conditions □ Vision Deficit □ Hearing Deficit □ Hx of Falls □ Hypotension □ CVD
□ Cognitive Deficit □ Wt. Loss □ Dehydration □ Hx CVA □ New Fx □ Parkinson's □ SOB
□ Hypertension □ Diabetes □ Neuropathy □ ↓ in ADL's □ Other (Specify): _____

Medications: □ Diuretic □ Antidepressant □ Hypnotic □ Anti-anxiety □ Antipsychotic
□ Cardiovascular □ Medication Chg. □ 9+ Medications □ Other (Specify): _____

Why Did This Incident Occur? (In Your Opinion): _____
_____

What Was Done Immediately? (To Prevent Reoccurence): _____
_____

Name of Person(s) Completing Report: _____
_____

REVIEW SIGNATURES:
Administrator _____ Date _____ DON _____ Date _____
QI _____ Date _____ Med. Director _____ Date _____
KDOA Workgroup05

Figure 1-1. Kansas Department of Aging Workgroup 05 Fall Incident Report Form (page 2 of 2).

Interview Time and Circumstances

Determining the best time to interview the patient will vary depending on
many factors and must be considered when scheduling the interview so as to
avoid patient fatigue, while maximizing the time needed to conduct the interview. If patients have pain associated with an injurious fall, conducting the
interview during pain-free moments is a priority. The patient in pain is likely
distracted and information may be withheld or forgotten altogether. Similarly,
the acutely disoriented, amnesic, or dazed patient is likely to be a poor histo-
rian until medically stable and speaking coherently. The nurse will need

to ascertain if the patient is capable of providing the needed information. Typically this will be determined by the nurse who has developed a relationship with the patient and knows the patient best.

Place of the Interview

Obtaining a fall-focused health history after a fall requires a private and comfortable environment for the patient. Once the patient has stabilized, this interview can take place in the patient's room or another private location in the home environment. The interviewer should avoid obtaining details about the fall event as the patient is lying on the floor. Rather, after the situation and patient have stabilized, conduct the interview in a private location on the unit they reside or in their home. There should be adequate lighting, comfortable seating, and a place for the nurse to record notes.

Special Considerations
What should I do if the patient appears seriously injured, and there is no time for an interview?

Depending on the nature of the injury and the medical stability of the patient after the fall, time is of the essence for obtaining critical life-saving information about the fall. In these cases, patient safety is a priority. A few situations occur, however, where standard interview protocol is deviated. This includes these three types of situations:

1. The patient sustained serious injury, such as head injury or a hip fracture and is bleeding profusely or experiencing extreme pain;

2. The patient who is lapsing into unconsciousness due to metabolic or hematological medical problems such as acute blood loss, profound dehydration, unstable vital signs, or hyperglycemia/hypoglycemia;

3. The case of the patient with unstable vital signs at the time of the fall:
   ► Apnea
   ► Tachypnea
   ► Bradycardia
   ► Hypo- or Hypertension
   ► Hypo- or Hyperthermia

In these cases, key symptoms and physical examination findings are urgently needed and must be obtained whenever the patient is encountered, including lying on the floor.

Note: Sudden change in mental status is the first step in determining if an urgent or life threatening injury may be in evolution or has occurred, such as a head injury.

What do I do if the patient seems confused or has poor fall recall?

The nurse should seek verification from other sources, such as healthcare providers who have cared for the patient, the patient's medical record or care plan, or the patient's family. Many times, verification of information from a reliable source can be handled on the telephone. Simply identify yourself and the nature of your inquiry about a prior fall (or falls) and the occurrence of any injury. Another useful source may be an eyewitness account of the fall.

What do I do if the patient seems puzzled or does not understand what I mean by a fall?

The term *fall* means different things to different people. In the healthcare setting, providers typically think of a person on the ground or floor or another lower surface. Several national organizations and professional societies have further defined what constitutes a "fall" for healthcare providers, but this perspective may not be shared by the patient. Consider the person who stumbles and trips, but catches themselves or eases themselves to their knee, is that a fall? Another example of where discrepancy in fall semantics may occur happens with children who fall. Fall events which occur in toddlerhood are "normal" milestones, provided there are no underlying pathological conditions linked to their fall. However, falls among children, as well as adults, may be symptomatic of an underlying pathological condition.

The words we use when discussing falls and the thoughts they evoke vary from patient to patient, according to age, gender, ethnic group, and culture. Depending on the native language spoken by the patient, the use of an illustration, picture, or hand gesture of a falling body can help the patient identify what the healthcare provider is referring to when asking about a fall event. Some providers point to the ground and ask "Have you fallen down to the floor or ground?" Many pictorial displays seen in the public domain appear to have some value in portraying images of falls.

General Factors for Consideration Influencing the Fall Health History

The principles of history-taking to elicit the fall health history take several factors into consideration. These include factors influencing communication of information by the patient, factors influencing the nurse's interviewing skills, knowledge, and attitude about falls, the relationship between the patient (interviewee) and the nurse (interviewer), the ability to communicate effectively, cultural awareness, and competence.

Each and every interviewer brings to the interview a unique set of values, beliefs, and attitudes, as well as perceptions about patient falls, including those they may have encountered with their own family members. Some of these perspectives can color the interview of the fall health history. Therefore interviewers must hold their personal perspectives separate and instead rely on recommended standard of care questions to elicit information. If the interviewer fails to keep the interview focused on the fall itself, extraneous conversation or missing information can occur.

Because falls and their prevention are unique and very personal experiences for the patient, it is important to identify each patient's own goals and plans for falls prevention and injury protection in addition to the provider's goals and plans.

Factors Influencing Communication of Information by the Patient

There are many factors influencing the patient's reception and expression of thoughts, all of which are subject to change depending on the medical stability of the patient. For example, a patient can be coherent and able to vividly describe the fall events verbally, and then hours later, lapse into a semi-conscious state due to a fall-related head injury, an event which the provider may have had no way to predict. The tendency to ask about falls retrospectively creates issues for populations of people at risk to fall and incur head injury who also have difficulty communicating or have cognitive impairment. Nurses can assess early in the healthcare encounter the patient's ability to learn, read, write, and understand. Simple commands like "Please write your name here on this piece of paper" can quickly ascertain: (a) receptivity of the command by the patient (i.e., that they can hear); and if performed accurately, (b) understanding by the patient of a basic one-step request or command. Additional factors which can influence verbal communication of the fall event include: hearing acuity, articulation of speech, phonation, level of alertness and native language. Care must be taken to ensure the patient has use of hearing aids and assistive devices for communication if needed, understands and can speak English, and is awake and sufficiently alert to participate in the interview.

Another critical factor influencing communication of information by the patient about the fall concerns the patient's memory of the fall. If a patient is falling multiple times, it is quite easy for them to mix up the events of one fall with those of another. Situating the fall within the context of time of day, what they were doing or wearing at the time of the fall or any particular major event, like a holiday or a birthday may remind the patient of the fall or trigger better recall. Referring back to the fall using these same identifiers is vital, in order to avoid mixing up fall one with fall two, and vice versa.

Learner Outcome 2: Incorporate historical medical information: The patient at risk for falling

Gathering the history for the patient at risk to fall, but who has never fallen.

Various age groups are susceptible to falls depending on their exposure to either extrinsic or intrinsic risk factors. Therefore a careful review of intrinsic and extrinsic risk factors is important during the annual medical encounter. A checklist can be created and administered annually to various age groups. Among children and teens, information about hazards in the environment are particularly important to review with parents and family caregivers. This is also an ideal time to elicit the patient's perception of their own fall risk. The following information can be included in the falls risk assessment.

The patient at risk for visual impairment (child or adult)

Visual impairment has long been associated with patient falls. Common questions the nurse will ask include:

- ► "How is your vision?"
- ► "Do you have any blurred vision?"
- ► "Do you use any reading aides or devices in school?"
- ► "When was the last date of visual acuity testing?"
- ► "When did you last have your vision tested?"
- ► "Do you use corrective lenses during recreation or sports?" or
- ► "Do you think it is important to wear corrective lenses during sports?"

The patient at risk for visual impairment (adult or older adult)

Patients with visual impairment may possess underlying medical problems such as a history of cataracts, prolonged use of steroids, macular degeneration, or retinal artery occlusion from carotid diseases which cause distortion of vision, retinal detachment, eye cancer, or other conditions causing impairment. Use of certain medications can also cause blurry vision symptoms, especially anti-cholinergic medications (for a more detailed listing, see the Beers criteria of inappropriate medication use). It is important to discover any history of eye surgery such as use of intra-ocular lens implantation for cataracts and to note if the patient uses corrective lenses and when their last ophthalmology visit occurred.

The evidence-based literature confirms that fall rates decline following correction of visual impairment, such as removal of cataracts. Hearing loss has also been implicated in the occurrence of falls. Among older adults, the American Geriatrics Task Force for Falls Prevention recommends annual screening in which questions about fall occurrences are asked. This is also an ideal time to elicit the patient's perception of their own fall risk and measures they have taken to reduce this risk. Common questions the nurse will ask include:

▶ "Overall, how is your vision?" "Do you think your vision is adequate?"

▶ "When was the last date of visual acuity testing?" (yearly screening is recommended)

▶ "Do you perceive the need to have your vision and hearing assessed yearly?"

▶ "Do you use corrective lenses and adaptive hearing deices during mobility?"

▶ "Do you have any blurred or double vision?" "Do you have any loss of vision in either eye?" "Do you use any reading aides or devices to function in your home?"

▶ "Have you had any eye surgery?" "Have you been diagnosed with glaucoma?"

▶ "Are there poorly lit areas in the stairwell in the home?"

▶ "Does the patient perceive that poor lighting might contribute to a fall?"

The patient at risk for gait or mobility impairment (child or adult)

Individuals of all ages have medical problems which can affect their gait, balance, and mobility. Common conditions seen in children and adults include muscular dystrophies, cerebral palsy, and joint diseases such as juvenile arthritis. Any one of these problems can impair gait, alter mobility or balance, and put the patient at risk for a fall. The nurse performing a fall risk assessment should elicit information about the patient's ability to walk. Does the patient have pain or weakness, does the patient use appropriate shoes or rely on adaptive aides to walk? Do they use any braces to assist with transfers? Depending on the age of the patient, do they perceive that wearing appropriate shoes while walking is necessary, as accidental falls can easily occur when walking barefooted? For younger children, parents and family caregivers should be asked about use of stair gates in the home and whether they perceive the need to ensure stairwell safety for their children.

The patient at risk for gait or mobility impairment (older adult)

Gait impairment is a broad classification of a disorder, influenced by many factors including medications, mental status, muscle strength, motion of the hips, knees, ankles, vision, vestibular input/hearing, and sensation/proprioception. Common issues seen in older adults likely to influence gait negatively include reduced muscle strength from arthritic joints, physical frailty wherein walking speed is reduced, sarcopenia associated with loss of muscle mass and strength, the hazards of immobility as well as use of inappropriate footwear. Elderly diabetics with peripheral neuropathy are also prone to gait disturbances related to sensing foot placement on the floor. Normal age-related changes in gait include decreased step height and speed of ambulation.

Gait impairments among older adults are most often multifactorial, and include: sensory deficits (visual, vestibular, somatosensory), neurodegenerative process (cortical, extrapyramidal motor, cerebellar), toxic (medications- or alcohol-related) and/or anxiety (primary or concerning falls) (Jahn et al., 2010). As it relates to falls, gait impairment is a classic risk factor implicated in production of falls in older adults (Stolze et al., 2004). Older adults may have chronic illnesses which directly impact mobility, gait, and balance.

Older patients with gait impairment may possess underlying medical problems such as a history of alcoholism, cerebellar disorders, stroke, Parkinson's Disease, secondary Parkinsonism (caused by medications), supranuclear palsy, or other conditions such as normal pressure hydrocephalus or a brain tumor. Other disorders lending to gait impairment may result from visual dysfunction and diseases resulting in decreased muscular strength of the ankles, hips, knees, legs, and shoulders. A prior hip fracture can result in muscular weakening of the hips. In many of the standard data sets, patient function is evaluated and coded according to protocol. The nurse should refer to these measures as well to verify recent patient performance.

Some of the more common diseases seen in this age group include lower extremity osteoarthritis (hip and knees) or rheumatoid arthritis which cause joint inflammation and destruction as well as produce symptoms of joint pain, tenderness, and fatigue. Another classic condition, polymyalgia rheumatica, affects the hip and shoulder joints producing inflammation and reduced joint mobility. Typically older adults with this condition will also experience difficulty such a pain or limitation with weight bearing activities. Another classic condition seen in this age group is osteoporosis which causes bone fragility. As bones become more brittle, they are susceptible to stress fractures from walking and patients may experience various types of low back pain as well. There are many circulatory and neurological problems which cause gait and mobility impairment. Many older adults have cardiovascular and circulatory diseases affecting the blood flow to the lower extremities. Those with coronary artery disease may experience angina with walking or leg extremity pain/claudication from poor circulation. One of the most prominent causes of death in older adults is stroke. A stroke can produce gait disturbances, hemiparesis, or complete paralysis. Vision, gait, balance, and ability to think are therefore affected to a degree depending on the nature and residual effects of the stroke. Because of these potential medical problems, it is recommended that the nurse ask about symptoms related to these conditions as well as the use of appropriate footwear and or assistive devices for mobility.

Common questions the nurse should ask the patient include:

- ► "Do you have any weakness in your legs with or without walking?"
- ► "How would you rate your walking ability today compared to a few months ago?"
- ► "Have you ever experienced your leg giving out or buckling while walking?" and
- ► "Do you use an assistive device to help you walk?"

Additionally, other important historical questions to inquire about from this age group include:

- ► "Do you experience any joint pain in your hips, knees, legs, shoulders?"
- ► "Do you feel weak in any particular muscle group?"
- ► "Are you affected by joint inflammation?"
- ► "Are you able to carry out your normal daily activities without limitation or pain in your joints?"
- ► "How do you perform exercise?" "Do you walk or swim for exercise?" "Do you use a bicycle or engage in Tai Chi?"
- ► "Do you use any braces or adaptive aides?"
- ► "How is your balance?" "Do you consistently walk into objects because of a loss of balance?"
- ► "What types of shoes do you wear for walking?"

Other questions for nurses to consider include: If mobility aides are used, are they sturdy? Does the patient know how to correctly use them? Does the patient perceive the need to wear adequate footwear to prevent slips or falls? If throw rugs are used on the landing surface, does the patient perceive throw rugs to be hazardous to their walking/potential to fall? Does the patient use handrails on the staircase? Are there grab bars near the toilet or in the shower? Does the patient perceive that using the grab bars can help steady balance and prevent falls?

The patient at risk for falls due to balance impairment (adult or older adult)

Balance disorders are a common and major cause of falls in older adult populations (Salzman, 2010). As noted by the National Institutes of Health (NIH, 2014), intact balance allows one to walk without staggering, to get up from a chair without falling, to climb stairs without tripping and to bend over without falling. The NIH further reports that in 2008 an estimated 14.8% of American adults (33.4 million) had a balance or dizziness problem during the past year (NIH, 2012).

Patients with balance impairment may possess underlying medical problems such as a history of hearing loss, labyrinthitis, Meniere's disease, inner ear infection, or circulatory disorders such as stroke. Some of the inner ear disorders can also result in dizziness, ear ringing, and room spinning (vertigo). A recent study by Agrawal (2014) found that patients with asymptomatic vestibular dysfunction were three times more likely to fall. Patients may also have a history of type 2 diabetes with peripheral neuropathy, orthostatic hypotension, dementia, normal pressure hydrocephalus, myelopathy, multiple sclerosis, or vertebrobasilar insufficiency. Medications, many of which are ototoxic can be implicated as well in disorders of equilibrium. Common questions the nurse should ask the patient include:

- ▶ "Do you have any loss of balance with standing up, sitting down or while walking?"
- ▶ "Do you feel unsteady on your feet?"
- ▶ "Do you experience dizziness or room spinning, and if so, have you fallen as a result?"
- ▶ "Do you experience ringing in your ears or loss of hearing?"

Other important information to discover includes the patient's perception of their balance and its relation to falls risk.

The patient at risk for falls due to use of high-risk medications (adult and older adult)

Research evidence shows the association between high-risk medications and risk to fall (Krauss et al., 2005; Leipzig, Cumming, & Tinetti, 1999). A more complete listing of various classifications of high-risk medications to avoid in older adults are included in the American Geriatrics Society *Updated Beers Criteria for Potentially Inappropriate Medication Use in Older Adults* (2012). High-risk medications include alcohol; prescription medications such as sedatives, hypnotics, anti-anxiety agents and narcotic analgesics; as well as illicit drug use. In the acute care setting, prescription medications may be administered orally, intramuscularly, or intravenously. In the latter methods, a more rapid response to the medication is likely. Due to the various illnesses affecting kidney and liver function, drugs can circulate in the system much longer than anticipated, posing hazardous adverse effects. In these cases, drug levels of an active metabolite can be assayed from a patient blood sample to check overall circulating levels for possible drug toxicity. Patients take prescription medications meant for pain for many reasons. One such medication is narcotic analgesia which can cause altered perception and sedation, even with one time or minimal use. Misuse or overuse of prescription drugs as well as use of illicit drugs such as marijuana, alone or combined with alcohol, may cause alterations in level of consciousness and produce hallucinations. Other illicit drugs such as hallucinogenic medications (LSD) and marijuana cause altered perception and alterations in level of consciousness. Some important issues to cover in the health history include:

► "What types of medications, prescription drugs, and illicit drugs, if any, is the patient taking?"

► "Do they stick to the prescription regimen or are they taking an overabundance of medications because of symptoms of anxiety, depression, or sleep disorders?"

► "Does the patient acknowledge the association between these medications and risk to fall?"

Learner Outcome 3: Incorporate historical medical information: The patient at risk for serious injury

Gathering the health history for the patient at risk for serious injury.

The prevention of serious injury due to a fall is a public health priority given the high incidence of fatal, and often preventable, falls. Serious, non-fatal injury as defined earlier includes events such as femur, pelvic or hip fracture, spinal fracture, internal bleeding, head trauma such as fractures to the orbit and skull, intracranial bleeding, and subdural hematoma. Many patients encountered in the healthcare setting suffer from diseases and conditions which place them at higher risk for serious injury. With early detection, the risk for serious injury can be lowered, as diseases can be treated earlier or interventions can be instituted to reduce trauma. The patient at risk for serious injury includes those patients with:

- ► Systemic diseases or conditions causing generalized weakness/debility (infection/sepsis),
- ► Osteoporosis,
- ► Altered mental status or states of delirium/sedation,
- ► Hypoglycemia,
- ► Patient taking blood thinners/anticoagulants,
- ► Blood disorders such as thrombocytopenia with low platelet counts or acute loss of blood or anemia, or
- ► Untreated orthostatic hypotension (OH), among other conditions.

The health history of the patients with OH or suspected OH

Orthostatic hypotension (OH) has been linked to patient falls among older adults (Gangavati et al., 2010; Ooi et al., 2000), and in the nursing home setting, OH coupled with symptoms of dizziness were predictive of falls (Duthie et al., 2007). Because OH can be easily detected, it is an essential component of the physical examination to isolate and manage so that falls can be prevented. We have noted in our prospective research study that despite OH protocol, OH determinations were often incomplete or absent in 41% (n=77) of all fall evaluations of elderly residents (Gray-Miceli, Ratcliffe, & Liu, 2012). This finding is surprising since the standard of care does require OH determination in falls evaluation (American Geriatrics/British Geriatrics Society, 2011; American Medical Directors Association, 1998; Chang et al., 2004).

OH is associated with any event causing a sudden reduction in blood volume such as acute loss of blood or dehydration. It is also associated with diseases such as diabetes mellitus and medications known to cause excessive diuresis. There are many other diseases and medications associated with or linked to OH. Patients with OH may possess underlying medical problems such as anemia, gastrointestinal bleeding, Parkinson's disease, type 2 diabetes, or dehydration. Patients may also take medications known to cause OH. Diuretics, laxatives, and agents which lower the blood volume are notorious culprits linked to OH. Classes of OH-associated medications are presented in Table 1-1. Drug-induced orthostatic hypotension is an infrequent adverse effect of medications such as alpha-1 blockers, with the first dose, adrenergic blockers, centrally acting drugs and others. See the classes of medications implicated in orthostatic hypotension (Table 1-1).

TABLE 1-1. **Classes of Medications Implicated in Orthostatic Hypotension (Schoenberger JA, 1991).**

Anti-hypertensives	Dopamine agonists
Diuretics	Phenothiazine
Adrenergic blockers	Tricyclic antidepressants
Vasodilator agents	Monoamine oxidase inhibitors
Anti-anginal agents	

Another significant condition for consideration in the evaluation of blood pressure and falls prevention among older adults is the occurrence of post-prandial hypotension. Post-prandial hypotension, a significant drop in blood pressure following a meal, is common in older hypertensive patients, although it is not fully understood (Jansen & Lipsitz, 1995).

The health history of the patient with mental status change

In the healthcare setting, the patient's mental status is subject to change depending on many interrelated factors. These factors are often physiologically based. Acute reasons can include events such as sudden hypoxia with dropping levels of oxygen saturation, drops in blood glucose, or profuse bleeding causing a rapid loss of blood volume. Both hypothermia and hyperthermia as well as bacterial infection, including sepsis, can quickly alter the patient's mental status. Following anesthesia, the patient is likely to experience drowsiness and prolonged periods of sedation or hypo-alertness. Other common causes of change in mental status include medication toxicity or use of any medication that causes adverse medication side effects resulting in drowsiness or sedation.

During the acute mental status change, the patient's level of consciousness and orientation to themselves (person), surroundings (place), or time is altered and inaccurate. Typically, this state of alertness fluctuates, where the patient can become drowsy and stuporous one moment, say at 7:00 am, and then at 8:40 am the same day, hyper-alert or restless. If the patient is engaged in an activity, they may execute poor judgment or be placed in unsafe situations due to their change in mental status. Thus in these situations falls are commonly encountered. Protecting patients from harm involves early recognition and reporting of the change in mental status. The term 'delirium' or 'acute confusion' is used when working with older adult populations to describe changes in mental status due to acute reasons.

The term *cognitive impairment* refers to long-standing changes in the brain resulting in impairment in the higher areas of cortical functioning. Common causes of cognitive impairment in older adults include dementia and traumatic brain injury, among others. Cognitive impairment is detected by a thorough medical evaluation, diagnostic studies, blood studies, and a classic historical account of events obtained by the examiner. Among other methods, the mental status examination is useful in the diagnostic assessment of cognitive impairment. Cognitive function as measured through mental status examinations has been associated with patient falls and recurrent falls, but has not been found to be predictive (Chen et al., 2012).

The health history of the patient taking high-risk medication implicated in falls risk and/or risk for non-spinal fracture

Central nervous system (CNS) medications are implicated in both falls risk and in risk for hip fracture injury. In prior seminal research studies of the Osteoporotic Fractures Research Group, the multivariate odds ratio of using certain CNS-active medications was computed, comparing users to non-users among older women to determine those at greatest risk for frequent falls (see Table 1-2; Ensrud et al., 2002) or at risk for non-spine fractures (see Table 1-3; Ensrud et al., 2003).

TABLE 1-2. **CNS Active Medications and Falls Risk in Older Women (Ensrud et al., 2002).**

Medication Class	Multivariate odds ratio with 95% Confidence Intervals (CI)
Antidepressants	1.54; (1.14-2.07)
SSRI	3.45; (1.89-6.30)
Tri-cyclic	1.28; (0.90-1.84)
Benzodiazepines	1.51; (1.14-2.01)
Short-acting	1.42; (0.98-2.04)
Long-acting	1.56; (1.00-2.43)
Anticonvulsants	2.56; (1.49-4.41)
Narcotics	0.99; (0.68-1.43)

TABLE 1-3. **CNS Active Medications and Risk for (Non-Spine) Fractures in Older Women (Ensrud et al., 2003).**

Medication Class	Multivariate hazard ratio with 95% Confidence Intervals (CI)
Narcotics	1.40; (1.06-1.83)
Antidepressants	1.65; (1.05-2.57)

Learner Outcome 4: Incorporate historical medical information: The patient who has fallen

Gathering the Post-Fall History

No matter the age of the patient being interviewed, the history obtained by the nurse should form a rich narrative so that the nurse can easily develop a mental image of the fall event which encompasses the four W's of the fall. *What, When, Where,* and *Why* did the fall occur? The fall onset in terms of timing, frequency and impact to the person, such as the presence of injury is also obtained. Because of the linkage of falls to underlying illnesses, additional questions about symptoms experienced with the fall must be addressed as well as the impact or outcome to the falling person. Details of how to conduct a health history to elicit the various dimensions of symptom presentation should be reviewed prior to startingthe interview, using available resources. Use of a stepwise approach is recommended for older adults with complex comorbidities for which deciphering various subtypes of falls requires additional information and analysis (Gray-Miceli et al., 2004). When the nurse can accurately replicate back to the patient the events leading to, during and following the fall, relevant symptoms, injury incurred and overall experience of the fall such as impact to the person, the initial fall health history is complete.

Obtaining The 4 W's of the Fall: What, When, Where, and Why

When eliciting the fall focused history from the patient, it is important to first ask for their account of the event. This is done so as to deter the patient from simply agreeing to another account such as that told by a witness. It also validates that you are interested in hearing and learning what the patient believes happened. Keep in mind that the patient account may be totally different than witness descriptions or the nurse's judgment of what happened. One way to lead the interview is to say, "tell me everything you can about your fall," or "describe everything you can recall about your fall, which occurred _____ (earlier today/an hour ago, etc.)". Using Table 1-4 as a rubric, the nurse can proceed to gather the *what, when, where,* and *why* of the fall.

- ► **What** elicits an overall description of what happened in the patients words which includes the activity at the time of the fall.
- ► **When** reveals calendar day, month, year and any associated holiday or event.
- ► **Where** reveals if the fall occurred indoors or outdoors. If inside, the specifics of the room and or use of equipment can help identify the where.
- ► **Why** helps the nurse understand the patient's thoughts about why the fall occurred.

TABLE 1-4. **Guidelines for Eliciting the *What, When, Where, Why* and *Impact* of the Fall.**

Questions of the Fall	Nurse's Statements	Descriptors of the Event/ Patient Responses
The *What*	Describe everything you can about what happened leading to your fall: *What* do you recall doing? What was your planned activity? Were you shopping? Leaning over? Walking? If the patient uses an assistive device, is it sturdy?	I was just standing there and then I fell. I was using the toilet and fell over when I stood up. I tripped over my cane.
The *When*	Describe *when* the fall occurred: Do you recall when the fall occurred? Was it during the night? During the day? Was the fall before or after Thanksgiving Holiday?	I fell in September. I fell close to Thanksgiving. I fell this morning at 6:00 am. I fell yesterday afternoon.
The *Where*	Describe *where* you were when the fall occurred? Were you in your home or outdoors? If inside, which room? Were you sitting down? Were you in bed? Were you standing up from a seated position?	I rolled over and fell out of my bed onto the floor. I fell while getting the mail outside in the front of the house. I fell down the steps.
The *Why*	*Why* do you think you fell?	I got dizzy standing up and I think I lost my balance and fell. I was reaching into the closet and fell into my clothes, landing on the floor. I was leaning on my cane and my knee buckled and I fell. I don't know why I fell.
Physical Impact from the Fall	Did you injure yourself? If yes, please describe: _____	I broke this bone here and was in a cast for a while.
Emotional Impact from the Fall	Did the fall impact on your emotions or overall sense of well-being? If yes, please describe: _____	I am really angry at myself for falling. I'm reluctant to walk around without that cane. The fall shook me up ... I don't know if I will ever get over it .... The fall changed my life.

In addition to the 4 W's, the nurse will need to learn more about the impact the fall has had, both physically and emotionally. A question to ask the patient is how the fall has affected their ability to stay independent in daily living. Here, the nurse may learn firsthand that the patient has developed a phobia or fear of falling or has limited their mobility outdoors. Fear of falling has been implicated in limitation of activities, mobility and ability to carry out activities in daily living (Vellas, Wayne, Romero, Baumgarner, & Garry, 1997; Lach, 2005; Friedman, Munoz, West, Reuben, & Fried, 2002). As well, a wide range of emotional responses to falls deemed serious to older adults has included angry, frustration, annoyance, and helplessness, among others (Gray-Miceli, 2001). All the information provided helps to inform a plan of care tailored to each individual.

Key Symptoms for Inquiry at the Time of the Patient Fall

Although the 4 W's (what, when, where and why) are asked post-fall, they do not get to how the patient was feeling at the time of the fall. Key symptoms associated with anticipated or unanticipated physiological falls and falls due to underlying pathological diseases range from drops in blood pressure from acute or chronic orthostatic hypotension to pathological reasons such as the sudden onset of a seizure or new hemorrhagic cerebrovascular stroke. Therefore it is important to always ask about key symptoms linked with falls which cause a clear alteration in physiological function. Generally the nurse can ask, "Can you tell me everything about how you were feeling at the time of your fall?" Following this, the nurse will need to ask a very specific set of questions in relation to the fall event. These questions are scattered throughout multiple systems of inquiry and need to be reported to the physician in the event that the fall is associated with one of these treatable events. Table 1-5 outlines the key symptoms to review with the patient and follow up with the physician in order to monitor the patient's health status.

Summary

Risk to fall, risk for serious injury, and actual falls all occur for several similar reasons. The likely or suspected risks and actual underlying causes can be identified when a focused fall health history and physical examination are performed. Use of the 4 W's as a framework can help in identifying the necessary elements of the history of a falling patient, while review of the classic fall risk factors, specific to various age groups can help detect those populations most susceptible to falls. There are many patient populations who have no identified risk to fall and who have never fallen, but will fall because they have an acute medical condition which may be missed if only a falls risk assessment tool is used. For this reason, the added value of the nurse's judgment is an essential component of determining risk to fall. Besides identifying patients' risks to fall, the fall history should include patients' perceived risks to fall and goals for reducing their risk.

TABLE 1-5. **Key Symptoms Arranged by System and Possible Conditions and Types of Fall.**

System and Symptoms	Possible Conditions	Possible Type of Fall
Behavioral Hunger, thirst Continuous wandering	Unmet physical needs Dementia with motor restlessness	Accidental Fall Environmental Fall Behavioral Fall Poor patient Safety Awareness Poor patient judgment
Cardiovascular system Lightheadedness Dizziness with standing Dizziness with head rotation Shortness of breath Syncope	Carotid stenosis, Cerebrovascular disease, Medications Orthostasis secondary to diabetes mellitus, volume depletion, PVD Carotid stenosis/ hypersensitivity Arrhythmia Neurological illnesses	Fall due to acute illness Fall due to chronic illness Anticipated physiological fall
Genitourinary Urinary urgency, frequency Urinary incontinence	Urinary tract infection Urinary tract infection	Fall due to acute illness Anticipated physiological
Neurological/ musculoskeletal Lower extremity numbness Bilateral Lower extremity weakness Unilateral Lower extremity weakness Loss of recall of the fall event Lower extremity joint pain Gait unsteadiness Sudden loss of balance	Neuropathy, diabetes mellitus, B12 deficiency, PVD (bilateral) Arthritis, disuse, thyroid disease, electrolyte imbalance CVA, arthritis Dementia Arthritis, sprain/strain, neuropathy Dementia, CVA, parkinsonism, foot problems Parkinson's disease, CVA	Fall due to acute illness Fall due to chronic illness Anticipated physiological
Pulmonary Dyspnea on exertion Lightheadedness with exertion	Emphysema, pneumonia Cardiovascular disease, anemia	Fall due to acute or chronic illness Anticipated physiological
General Sudden weakness Fatigue Focal pain Dizziness with head movement	Frailty, disuse, anemia Severe anemia, CHF, infection Bone fracture, soft tissue injury Labyrinthitis, cervical arthritis	Fall due to acute or chronic illness Anticipated physiological

References

American Geriatrics Society and British Geriatrics Society. (2011). Algorithim available at: http://www.medcats.com/FALLS/frameset.htm

American Geriatrics Society and British Geriatrics Society Panel on Prevention of Falls in Older Persons. (2011). Summary of the updated American Geriatrics Society/British Geriatrics Society clinical practice guideline for prevention of falls in older persons. *J Am Geriatric Soc., 59*(1), 148–57.

American Geriatrics Society Updated Beers Criteria for Potentially In Appropriate Medication Use in Older Adults. JAGS. doi: 10.1111/j.1532-5415.2012.03923.x Available at: http://www.americangeriatrics.org/files/documents/beers/2012BeersCriteria_JAGS.pdf

Chang, J. T., Morton, S. C., Rubenstein, L. Z., et al. (2004). Interventions for the prevention of falls in older adults: Systematic review and meta-analysis of randomized clinical trials. *British Medical Journal 20,* 328 (7441), 680.

Chen, T. Y., Peronto, C. L., & Edwards, J. D. (2012). Cognitive function as a prospective predictor of falls. (First published online: August 3, 2012.) *Journal of Gerontology, Series B: Psychological Sciences and Social Sciences, 67*(6), 720–728. doi: 10.1093/geronb/gbs052

Department of Health and Human Services, Office of the Inspector General. (2012). Hospital incident reporting systems do not capture most patient harm. January. Publication OEI-06-09-00091. Available at http://oig.hhs.gov/oei/reports/oei-06-09-00091.pdf

Duthie, E. H., Katz, P. R., & Malone, M. L. (2007). *Practice of Geriatrics.* 4th ed. Philadelphia, PA: Saunders-Elsevier.

Ensrud, K. E., Blackwell, T. L., Mangione, C. M., et al. (2002). Central nervous system—active medications and risk for falls in older women. *Journal of the American Geriatric Society, 50*(10), 1629–37.

Ensrud, K. E., Blackwell, T. L., Mangione, C.M., et al. (2003). *Annals of Internal Medicine, 163*(8), 949–57.

Friedman, S. M., Munoz, B., West, S. K., Rubin, G. S., & Fried, L. P. (2002). Falls and fear of falling: Which comes first? A longitudinal prediction model suggests strategies for primary and secondary prevention. *Journal of the American Geriatrics Society 50*(8), 1329–1335.

Gangavati, A., Hajjar, I., Quach, L., Jones, R. N., Kiely, D. K., Gagnon, P., & Lipsitz, L. A. (2011). Hypertension, orthostatic hypotension, and the risk of falls in a community-dwelling elderly population: The maintenance of balance, independent living, intellect, and zest in the elderly of Boston study. *Journal of the American Geriatrics Society, 59*(3), 383–389.

Gray-Miceli, D. (2001). A Phenomenological study of the meaning of serious falls to older adults. Widener University, Doctoral Dissertation. UMI Microform No: 3005877.

Gray-Miceli, D., Johnson, J. C., & Strumpf, N. E. 2005. A Stepwise approach to comprehensive post-fall assessment. *Annals of Long-Term Care and Aging 13*(12), 16–24.

Gray-Miceli, D., Ratcliffe, S. J., Liu, S., Wantland, D., Johnson, J. (2012). Orthostatic hypotension in older nursing home residents who fall: Are they dizzy? *Clinical Nursing Research, 21*(1), 64–78. doi: 10.1177/1054773811434045

Jansen, R. W., & Lipsitz, L. A. (1995). Postprandial hypotension: epidemiology, pathophysiology, and clinical management. *Annals of Internal Medicine, 122*(4), 286–295.

Klaus J. K., Andreas Z. A., & Schniepp, R. (2010). Gait disturbances in old age: Classification, diagnosis, and treatment from a neurological perspective. *Deutsches Ärzteblatt International, 107*(17), 306–316. doi: 10.3238/arztebl.2010.0306

Krauss, M. J., Evanoff, B., Hitcho, E., Ngugi, K. E., Dunagan, W. C., Fischer, I., Birge, S., Johnson, S., Costantinou, E., & Fraser, V. J. (2005). A Case-control Study of Patient, Medication, and Care-related Risk Factors for Inpatient Falls. *J Gen Intern Med., 20*(2), 116–122. doi: 10.1111/j.1525-1497.2005.40171.x

Leipzig, R. M., Cumming, R. G., & Tinetti, M. E. (1999). Drugs and falls in older people: A systematic review and meta-analysis, Part I. Psycho-tropic drugs. *Journal of the American Geriatrics Society, 47*, 30–39.

Leipzig, R. M., Cumming, R. G., & Tinetti, M. E. (1999). Drugs and falls in older people: A systematic review and meta-analysis, Part II. Cardiac and analgesic drugs. *Journal of the American Geriatrics Society, 47*, 40–50.

Lach, H. W. (2005). Incidence and risk factors for developing fear of falling in older adults. *Public Health Nursing 22*(1), 45–52.

Ooi, W. L., Barrett, S., Hossain, M., & Lipsitz, L. A. (2000). The association between orthostatic hypotension and recurrent falls in nursing home residents. *The American Journal of Medicine, 108*(2), 106–111.

National Institutes of Health. (2012). NIH Senior Health. *Balance problem*s. Retrieved from http://nihseniorhealth.gov/balanceproblems/aboutbalanceproblems/01.html

Salzman, B. (2010). Gait and balance disorders in older adults. *American Family Physician, 82*(1), 61–8.

Schoenberger, J. A. (1991). Drug-induced orthostatic hypotension. *Drug Safety, 6*(6), 402–7.

Stolze, H., Klebe, S., Zechlin, C., et al. (2004). Falls in frequent neurological diseases: Prevalence, risk factors and aetiology. *Journal of Neurology, 251*(1), 79–84.

Vellas, B. J., Wayne, S. J., Romero, L. J., Baumgarner, R. N., & Garry, P. J. (1997). Fear of falling and restriction of mobility in elderly fallers. *Age and Ageing, 26*: 189–193.

Useful Web-based Resources

Agency for Healthcare Research and Quality (AHRQ) National Guideline Clearinghouse. Guideline Summary NGC-9721. Fall Prevention.

American Geriatrics Society. (2010). www.americangeriatrics.org/health_care_professionals/clinical_practice/clinical_guidelines_recommendations/2010.

American Geriatrics Society and British Geriatrics Society. (2010). AGS/BGS Clinical Practice Guidelines: Prevention of Falls in Older Persons. New York: NY.

Hartford Institute for Geriatric Nursing: Consult Geri RN: Beers Criteria ConsultgeriRN.org/topics/Beers_critieria/want_to_know_more

Step 2. Conducting a Fall-Focused Physical Assessment

Overview

The physical assessment is a critical component of any falls risk analysis or post-fall evaluation. It provides an opportunity for the nurse to detect abnormalities such as injury or hypotension so that further individualized treatment and plans of care can be implemented. Early resolution of these abnormalities can reduce falls risk factors and subsequent recurrent falls.

In order to properly execute the physical assessment, the nurse will need to assemble several items such as a thermometer, a watch with a second hand, stethoscope, pen light, blank paper and pen, blood pressure cuff, and the patient's medical record for recording all physical findings. In order to assess the musculoskeletal and neurological systems fully, additional training may be needed as well as knowledge of how to use standard assessment tools. For this reason, referral to interprofessional specialists such as physical or occupational therapists or geriatricians is warranted. Some of the more commonly used assessment tools will be highlighted in this chapter.

Prior to initiating the physical assessment, the patient will need to be in a comfortable position in a private location with adequate lighting. There should be a straight back chair with armrests, a bed which can be placed in high and low positions, and a bedside stand for the patient to use. Ideally, patients should be pain free, have their corrective lenses and hearing aide available if customarily used, wear shoes normally worn for ambulation, and wear a gown. The entire physical examination, minus gait and ambulation assessments, can take place with the patient in bed, should they be immobile. Patients need to be informed of the purpose of the physical assessment and the estimated time to complete the examination. Once the examination is complete, the patient is made aware of pertinent findings for which additional monitoring is warranted. Important physical examination findings are reviewed so that the patient becomes engaged in the post-fall evaluation process.

Guidelines for items to include in the post-fall evaluation are recommended in the prevailing clinical practice guidelines set forth by national organizations, professional societies and current evidence-based practice (AHRQ, National Clearinghouse Clinical Practice Guidelines). For community-dwelling older adults, the American Geriatrics Society algorithm for physical assessment is included in the ten-step process following the fall history.

Broad Public Health Service Objective: Monitor Health Status to Identify and Solve Community Problems

Educational Learner Outcomes

At the conclusion of the chapter, the learner should be able to:

► Differentiate between the necessary elements of a falls risk assessment versus a comprehensive post-fall analysis;

► Recognize fall-related injuries which can be detected through a comprehensive post-fall assessment;

► Perform a correct physical assessment for detecting orthostatic hypotension; and

► Conduct and interpret the findings from the "Timed Get Up and Go" (TUG) test alongside occupational or physical therapists.

Learner Outcome 1. Falls Risk Assessment, Post-Fall Analysis, and Post-Fall Assessment

Learner Outcome 1A. Differentiate the necessary elements of a falls risk assessment versus a comprehensive post-fall analysis.

Learner Outcome 1B. Recognize fall-related injuries that can be detected through a comprehensive post-fall assessment.

Components of the physical examination for the fall risk assessment and comprehensive post-fall assessment

Table 2-1 details the components of the physical examination that should follow a fall history in order to begin to identify actual fall risk factors. The fall risk analysis is the preferred method for screening a patient for risk factors to fall, while a comprehensive post-fall evaluation includes both the fall risk assessment and any additional details depending on the patient population surveyed. These findings are then discussed with interdisciplinary teams to identify which factors are modifiable and which factors are non-modifiable so that the type of fall most likely to occur can be determined and the plan of care set in motion.

Some of the common physical impairments associated with falls are presented in this chapter (visual, gait and balance impairment, cognitive impairment, and orthostatic hypotension). Within these physical impairments, three areas are discussed:

▶ How do you determine if the impairment is present?

▶ What are useful screening measures to validate the impairment by the nurse, occupational therapist or physical therapist?

▶ What are some modifications to the assessment that will ensure patient safety?

The following section on physical examination follows content provided in Table 2-1.

TABLE 2-1. Components of the Physical Examination for the Comprehensive Fall Risk Assessment (Never Fallen) and the Comprehensive Post-Fall Assessment (Recent Fall).

Examination Component	Associated Learner Outcome	Content typically included on Fall Risk Assessment Tool? (Yes/No)	Content typically included on Comprehensive Post-Fall Evaluation Tool? (Yes/No)
Vital signs		Yes	Yes
Orthostatic hypotension		Depends on the tool used	Yes
Visual acuity		Yes	Yes
Hearing		No	Yes
Head/neck condition		No	Yes
Pupil assessment		No	Yes
Cardiovascular: Heart rate		No	Yes
Pulmonary: Lungs		No	Yes
Gastrointestinal/rectal		No	Yes
Musculoskeletal: Spine, weight-bearing joints, tandem walking; Gait; straight leg raising; Gait impairment		Depends on measures used; typically includes the Timed "Get Up and Go" test	Yes
Footwear		No	No
Neurological: Cranial nerves; Deep tendon reflexes (DTR); Balance impairment		Depends on tool used	Yes
Cognitive assessment using screening measures		Possibly	Yes

Vital Signs

The physical assessment must always include measurement of the patient's vital signs. This includes assessment of pain as the fifth vital sign. Patients should not be in pain prior to a fall. Assessing pain and providing relief is critical before beginning the examination. Pain can elevate heart rate and blood pressure; therefore pain should be noted and treated. Equally important, post-fall pain in the spine, groin or hip area can be an early sign of a serious injury, such as vertebral fracture, hip fracture, or pelvic fracture. If this pain is new post-fall, additional evaluation for injury is warranted.

Temperature can be assessed by several routes, but ultimately the route chosen will depend upon the patient's current situation. Elevations in temperature can result in the patient feeling weak or tired, factors which are implicated in falls. Low body temperatures, under 97 degrees Fahrenheit, indicate hypothermia and require reporting to the physician for further evaluation in addition to re-warming the patient. Blood pressure readings should be evaluated by the same examiner with the patient resting in a seated position. Orthostatic hypotension assessment requires the patient to stand with assistance from the examiner as the blood pressure is taken a second time. For more detail on assessment of orthostatic hypotension, see the section below. Respiratory rate is an important vital sign which can indicate an underlying infection or other serious illness. Traditionally respiratory rate is counted for one minute; the quality of the respirations is noted as well.

Learner Outcome 2: Physical Assessment for Orthostatic Hypotension

Perform a correct physical assessment for detecting orthostatic hypotension (OH).

The Patient at Risk for OH or with OH

Orthostatic hypotension (OH) is defined as a drop in the systolic and/or diastolic blood pressure within three minutes of a change in position (Consensus Committee of the American Autonomic Society & The American Academy of Neurology, 1996). Traditionally, three measures are obtained by the nurse or examiner from the same arm of the patient: the blood pressure when supine (lying down), sitting, and standing. When a drop of 20 mmHg occurs in the systolic reading or a drop in the diastolic reading of 10 mmHg or more occurs, the diagnosis of OH is made.

The nurse may suspect OH should the patient stand from a seated position and suddenly appear weak, lose balance, or complain of dizziness. The traditional hallmark sign of OH is patient complaints of lightheadedness and/or dizziness. However, in our study of elderly individuals who fell with OH, patients' complaints of loss of balance were voiced instead, with no complaints of dizziness (Gray-Miceli et al., 2012). These findings speak to asymptomatic OH, which has also been found by research conducted by Bradley and Davies (2003).

Special Consideration for Patients at Risk for OH or with OH

Although nurses expect patients with OH to demonstrate the classic signs of dizziness alongside drops in blood pressure upon standing, this is not always the case. Asymptomatic OH can occur, prompting nurses to be hyper-vigilant in detecting OH through regular OH blood pressure determinations among persons who fall.

Determining if OH is Present

Determining if the patient has OH requires careful determination of blood pressure in three positions.

It is ideal to take the blood pressure in the same arm with the patient lying, sitting, and then standing; however, without the assistance of another person, for instance provision of contact guarding or use of appropriate tilt tables, this is not often as easy as it may appear.

Special Considerations for Determining if OH is Present in Frail, Debilitated, or Weakened Patients
Frail, debilitated, or weakened patients

In the situation where the nurse is attempting to check the OH blood pressures in frail, debilitated or weakened individuals, he or she must be aware that when they attempt to sit or stand the patient up, the patient may collapse. For this reason, it is advisable to:

- Constantly speak to the patient to find out how they are feeling on a moment-to-moment basis during the OH assessment;
- Have at least one other person assisting you to provide contact guarding of the patient; and/or
- Perform a modified assessment of OH.

Modifications in the assessment to ensure patient safety: Patient supine (sitting)

Performing a modified assessment of OH is a safety precaution where the OH blood pressure readings are only taken with the patient lying supine to a sitting position. For example, Figure 2-1 illustrates a frail elderly woman whose blood pressure was 110/60 supine and 90/50 sitting. In the case of profound electrolyte imbalances caused by loss of blood or dehydration, OH may exist from supine to sitting position, and thus standing the patient is not necessary, as the criteria has already been met.

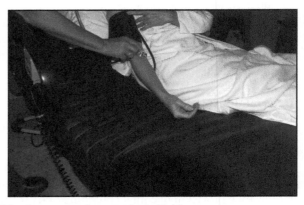

Figure 2-1. Assessment of OH blood pressure using a graduated table.

Use of specialized tables

Figure 2-2 illustrates a table which is low to the floor and can be placed into various positions to assess for OH.

Documentation of OH

It is very important to document the OH findings in the patient's vital sign record, and in the medical record, for providers to review as well as to communicate significant findings to providers immediately. Traditionally physician's orders will be written to obtain OH readings over three different occasions and to notify the provider of the findings so that treatment can be instituted. An assessment form is available through the CDC's STEADI toolkit, but traditionally the patient's vital sign record is where the OH readings are documented.

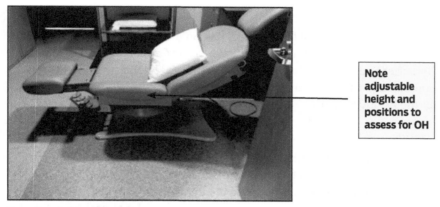

Note adjustable height and positions to assess for OH

Figure 2-2. Adjustable table.

Visual Acuity

The Patient at Risk for or with Visual Impairment
Eliciting visual impairment

Traditionally with the patient seated, the nurse examiner will test for visual acuity using a handheld eye chart, held 14 inches away from the patient. The patient's vision can be assessed both with and without corrective lenses. With the patient's eye glasses or contact lenses intact, monocular vision can be assessed by asking the patient "to cover the right eye and with the left eye to read the smallest print they can see on the handheld card." Corresponding numbers will indicate if the line the person can correctly visualize is 20/20 or 20/40. Once the left eye is assessed, monocular vision in the right eye is assessed by covering the opposite (left) eye. Other quick measures to assess gross binocular visual acuity are to ask the patient if they can read a passage from a magazine or other printed material out loud. This gives the nurse an idea if the patient can see well enough to read printed materials.

Ask the patient to cover one eye, or cover the eye by placing your hand over the patient's right eye; have the patient look at your nose and ask them whether they can see your entire face or not. The entire field of vision should be intact. Conditions associated with a loss of vision include macular degeneration or the presence of a cataract and can result in loss of a visual field. Alternatively, the patient can be asked with one eye covered if they see your fingers wiggling, as you move your fingers through the fields of gaze.

Asking the patient to cover their eye and testing for light perception is also relevant. Persons who are blind may be unable to perceive light; this has numerous safety implications for physical functioning in their environment.

Useful screening measures

Patients with a history of falls and any person over the age of 65 should undergo yearly ophthalmology evaluation as recommended by the American Geriatrics Society (AGS/BGS, 2011). The handheld Snellen eye chart can be purchased in medical–surgical supply stores or at university campus centers for the health sciences.

Hearing

Traditionally hearing acuity is assessed as part of Cranial Nerve XIII testing. Hearing impairment can be easily assessed by having the patient occlude one ear and having the examiner stand to the opposite side of the occluded ear and whisper a word or numbers. This is repeated on the opposite ear. Results to this whisper test can then be used in the overall determination of risk to fall. Other important observations are the presence of mechanical obstruction from accumulated cerumen (earwax) or the presence of sensorineural hearing loss. Performance of an audiometry exam is beyond the scope for the registered nurse charged with assessing the patient. However, referral to an interdisciplinary team member such as an audiologist can provide a rather quick assessment for presbycusis, a type of age-related hearing loss. Presbycusis is a high tone frequency hearing loss which, when assessed, can aid medical professionals in the overall determination of risk to fall.

Head and neck

The nurse carefully inspects the head for any signs of cranial trauma or bulging. Any lacerations or old bruises should be noted. The neck examination centers on gentle range of motion of the cervical spine. Documentation of any abnormalities, discoloration such as bruises, hematomas, or open lacerations are made on the diagram of the human head. The location of the laceration or hematoma is described in millimeters.

Modifications in the assessment to ensure patient safety

Care needs to be taken when passively moving the older adult's neck, or palpating the neck so as to avoid occlusion of the carotid arteries. A condition called carotid hypersensitivity has been noted in older adults and can result in a temporary loss of blood flow if the arteries are occluded by undue force from the examiner's hand.

Pupil assessment

Using a pen light, the nurse carefully assesses the size (diameter) and symmetry of the pupil. Note that older adults may have an asymmetrical pupil due to a prior cataract surgery. Pupils should respond equally and briskly to light and accommodation. Pupil assessment is traditionally covered in assessment of the cranial nerves. Pupil assessment is very important especially in cases where head injury is suspected. As part of the Glasgow Coma Scale, pupil size, symmetry, and reactivity to light and accommodation are monitored closely and abnormalities of new onset are quickly acted upon.

Cardiovascular Assessment

Using inspection, auscultation, palpation, and percussion, the nurse can quickly assess the cardiovascular system. Existence of bruits can be noted in any of the arteries using the bell of the stethoscope. Careful auscultation over the carotid artery can detect a unilateral or bilateral bruit. Bruits are important clinical findings especially in the case where a fall is believed to be due to an acute or chronic medical condition such as carotid stenosis. The apex and the base of the heart are examined using auscultation to detect any murmurs. Aortic stenosis is a clinical condition that can be detected by auscultation over the aortic valve. The triad of symptoms associated with aortic stenosis of a critical or advanced nature includes syncope, chest pain or shortness of breath, and heart failure. Listening over the point of maximal impulse (PMI) for one minute, the nurse notes the rate and rhythm of the heart. If arrhythmias are suspected, electrocardiograms are performed to detect atrial or ventricular arrhythmias or various types of heart block. The arteries of the lower extremities are also examined and inspected for bruits. Color and skin temperature and palpation for the presence of pulses in the femoral, post-popliteal, post-tibialis and dorsalis pedis areas are clinically relevant for the detection of arterial insufficiency or occlusion.

Pulmonary System

Patients at risk for falling include those who have pulmonary infections and/or end-stage heart failure. Careful auscultation of the lungs can detect rales, rhonchi, or wheezes which could be indicative of a mass of fluid or obstruction of airflow commonly occurring with acute pneumonia, bronchitis or congestive heart failure. Inspection and palpation of the rib cage is also very important; here, any point of tenderness over the rib cage or sternum could indicate a fractured rib. Any splinting of inspiration by the patient or any evidence of skin discoloration and bruising should be carefully noted and reported to the physician.

Modifications in the Assessment to Ensure Patient Safety

Care needs to be taken by the examiner when palpating the rib cage or assessing for pulmonary excursion of a frail, debilitated or weakened patient, who may have osteoporosis and an existing rib cage fracture.

Gastrointestinal System

Beginning with an assessment of oral mucosa for moistness, nurses can detect early signs of dehydration which can be implicated in falls risk. Having the patient stick out their tongue and noting the degree of moistness is important. With the patient supine, the abdominal cavity is also examined to determine the presence or absence of any acute trauma or injury. By gentle palpation and inspection, signs of trauma can be detected. As well, auscultation should produce equal bowel sound throughout all four quadrants. There should be no bruising or sings of abdominal swelling, which could indicate fluid in the abdomen. If trauma or fluid is suspected, the physician should be contacted immediately or, if the physician is unavailable, the patient should be moved to the local emergency department for further assessment.

Modifications in the Assessment to Ensure Patient Safety

During the abdominal examination, the examiner may suspect active gastrointestinal bleeding. Gastrointestinal bleeding can be the end product of trauma to the abdominal cavity from a fall or a precursor to a fall. In either event, should the patient loose blood volume and become hypotensive, the examiner will need to raise the side rails, elevate both lower extremities, and notify the physician immediately. A rectal examination assessing for the presence of blood is frequently warranted to eliminate this possibility. If the physician is unavailable, the patient is moved to the local emergency department for further assessment.

Musculoskeletal System

The Patient at Risk for or with Gait Impairment

The nurse assesses the musculoskeletal system, noting strength of upper and lower extremities among the major muscle groups. With the patient supine in bed, they can be asked to raise one leg at a time. The nurse should note their range of motion and if movements produce any pain. Pain and limitation of motion are early signs of a fractured extremity. Gait and footwear are also included as part of the musculoskeletal assessment.

Gait has been defined as "moving your center of gravity from one place to another in a safe and energy-efficient manner" (Inman, 1981). Traditionally, the clinical assessment of gait by nurses involves a carefully observation of the patient walking across the room from one point to another. Nurses stand behind the person to determine if their walking path is in a straight line or if it is deviated, also noting step height and speed. There is, however, much more involved in gait analysis and pinpointing the problem area than presented in this simplified maneuver for assessing a person's ability to walk. Full gait analysis uses dynamic electromyogram monitoring, force plates (kinetics), video analysis, and electrogoniometers in supervised settings by rehabilitation experts.

Characteristics of gait include walking speed, cadence, center of gravity, step length, and base of support. According to Inman (1981), the gait cycle involves two phases: one related to the stance and stability with weight transfer (this constitutes up to 60% of the cycle of gait), and the other with the swing of the limb and advancement of the limb (this constitutes about 40% of the gait cycle).

Determining if a Gait Impairment is Present

The professional nurse can independently determine whether the patient's gait is grossly normal. However, because of a lack of specialty training, the nurse is not expected to be able to identify either the origin or the type of gait abnormality that may exist should one be identified. Hence, referral to a falls clinic, geriatrician, physiatrist, neurologist or advanced practice nurse specializing in falls prevention or rehabilitation would be warranted for this determination.

Observations of Patient Gait

Asking the patient to rise from a seated position and walk across the room will provide many important aspects of the gait assessment. Using a chair with arm rests provides a greater degree of safety to assume a standing position (see Figure 2-3) than using a chair which has no supportive arm rests (see Figure 2-4). Note if the patient pushes his or her self up with both arms to a standing position. This can be a sign of hip weakness.

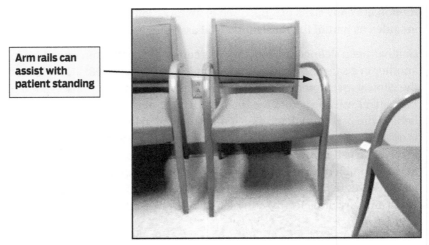

Arm rails can
assist with
patient standing

**Figure 2-3. Supportive straight back chair from which
the patient can rise to a standing position.**

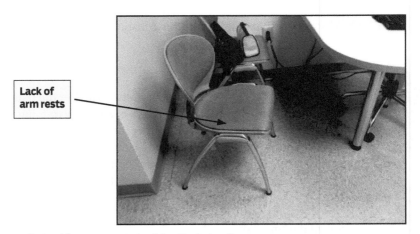

Lack of
arm rests

Figure 2-4. Chair with no arm rests to aid patient standing.

Patient Safety Issues

Nurses must use their best judgment in determining the degree of assistance
or supervision needed by patients getting in and out of chairs. Decisions
made are subject to change, depending on the medical stability of the patient.
Referring to a recent functional assessment, or performing one, identifies
areas of dependency and independence in basic skills related to transferring,
walking, dressing, bathing or toileting. Typically, functional assessment is
performed upon admission to a facility, on change in the level of care, and

following a patient fall. Employers must develop protocols and have educational training in place for healthcare workers so that patient safety and safe mobility is not compromised. (Standard 2 in Gallagher, 2013; pp. 26–27).

Special Considerations

The standard assessments performed by the nurse to determine muscular strength and joint range of motion will help identify joint contracture or focal muscle weakness. An integral component of the gait assessment is attention to the lower extremities for identification of hip, knee, or ankle muscle weakness. All of these muscles work synergistically to keep the patient upright and walking.

The nurse will note the patient's walking speed, any deviation to the side as they walk a straight line, cadence (normally 80 steps per minute), step length (15 inches on average), and step height. Situations which cause decreased step height include the type of shoe worn as well as medical issues such as the presence of dementia or Parkinson's Disease. The nurse should note if the patient leans to one side or another. Leaning suggests a possible muscle weakness in the lower extremities or a cerebral deficit as in the case of a stroke or cerebellar disorder.

Modifications in the Assessment to Ensure Patient Safety

As the gait assessment is performed, the examiner may note the patient is unsteady.

If the patient is unsteady, they may require arm-in-arm assistance from the nurse or staff or need to use an assistive device to maintain upright balance or assist with weight bearing. If the nurse is unsure of the patient's ability to ambulate, it is always safest to have a second person available to assist the patient while the nurse observes to assess gait. For patient safety reasons, another option is to defer this part of the examination altogether until a skilled expert can assess the patient.

Should an older adult patient over age 65 living in the community demonstrate a gait impairment or unsteadiness, a comprehensive assessment of the fall or a fall evaluation by a trained specialist is warranted (American Geriatrics Society, Falls Prevention, 2011; see www.medcats.com/FALLS/frameset.htm).

Other Considerations

Footwear

Footwear is an essential part of the patient's "ability to walk." Falls occur when patients slip on floor surfaces when in stockings or bare feet. Ideally shoes should have a rubber sole, a wedge heel, and good ankle support. The use of Velcro fasteners may be preferable to shoelaces, which if untied can contribute to tripping while walking. Overall, the base of support is critical to walking, and wearing inappropriate shoes can alter the base of support and disrupt balance. Figure 2-5 illustrates appropriate shoes for older adults.

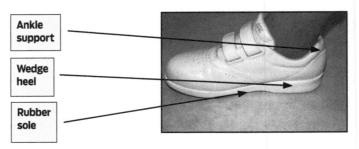

Figure 2-5. Appropriate shoes for older adults.

Modifications in the assessment to ensure patient safety

In order to ensure patient safety while assessing gait, it is never advisable to assess or observe the patient ambulate in their stockings or bare feet. In addition, slippers that do not have rubber soles or support for the ankle can lead to a patient slipping and falling. Before assisting the patient to ambulate so that gait can be assessed, it is therefore advisable that shoes be put on the patient's feet before getting out of bed.

Shoulder, Arm, and Hand Strength

Should the patient have trouble with walking, it is likely they will use an assistive device to aid with mobility. To use this device will require upper extremity shoulder, arm, and hand strength. The nurse will also need to assess the upper extremities for strength and assess the patient's ability to grip the assistive device.

Learner Outcome 3. Interprofessional Timed Up and Go (TUG) test

Conduct and interpret findings from the "Timed Get Up and Go" (TUG) test along with occupational or physical therapists.

Useful Screening Measures Conducted by Nurses and Occupational and Physical Therapists

Because of the nurse's schedule and staffing issues, it may not always be feasible for nurses to perform assessments of strength, gait, or balance. Occupational and physical therapists are specially trained to perform these assessments, typically with the assistance of others. In therapy departments, both have access to equipment specially designed for patients with impairments in gait or balance, providing some degree of patient safety during these tests and transfer maneuvers. For instance, there is ample floor and chair padding as well as staff assigned to each patient so that injury risk is minimized. So, when in doubt, it is best to defer to these professionals or to coordinate the nursing and the occupational/physical therapy assessment jointly.

The TUG and the Functional Gait Assessment have been used to assess for gait and balance impairment by occupational and physical therapists. Both tools are reliable and valid measures. If the nurse is unfamiliar with the TUG or has never performed the TUG assessment, it is recommended the nurse perform the TUG alongside the therapist. The TUG test is a simple test in which the patient stands up from a chair, walks 10 feet, turns around, walks back and sits in the chair once again. Normally it will take a patient less than 10 seconds to complete the task and this finding indicates they have no impairment in mobility status and likely need no further assessment. However, because the time taken to perform the test is scored, various scores in time coupled with the patients mobility status indicate the risk for falling, the need for further assessment, and the type of intervention most useful. As such, patients with TUG scores greater than 30 seconds indicate mobility impairment, high risk for falls and require additional assessment and intervention. Overall, the TUG test has sensitivity from 54–87% and specificity up to 87%, correlating with impairment in activities of daily living (Podsiadlo, 1991). An instructional video on how to administer the TUG is available in the STEADI tool kit, courtesy of the Centers for Disease Control (www.cdc.gov/homeandrecreationalsafety/Falls/steadi/videos.html).

The Functional Gait Assessment is more a detailed assessment for postural stability during walking tasks, and is best administered by a trained occupational or physical therapist in a controlled setting such as a therapy department.

Neurological Assessment: Cranial Nerves, Deep Tendon Reflexes, and the Patient At Risk for or with Balance Impairment

The nurse assesses the patient's cranial nerves following customary procedures. Any new unilateral findings are important to note and report to the physician. Many times, a recent stroke is detected as a reason for a fall when the patient is suddenly found to have a facial drop or a hemi-paresis of new onset. Asking the patient to smile can elicit a facial drop. In addition, asking the patient to extend their arms in front of their body with eyes closed can easily detect a pronator drift or upper extremity paresis. Deep tendon reflexes should also be assessed and should be symmetrical. Note there is a tendency for older adults to have decreased DTR's but not absent DTRs. The plantar response is also noted, and if abnormal it can indicate a new stroke. New neurological findings must be reported immediately to the physician.

There are many types of balance we observe among patients in the healthcare setting. Examples include the patient sitting balanced in a chair or on the edge of a bed and their ability to stand upright (static balance). When assessing for gait impairment and observing the patient walk, we are also simultaneously observing dynamic balance. Dynamic balance reflects one's ability to adjust and maintain an upright posture without falling over and despite being displaced. Patients with balance impairment often report symptoms of loss of balance or unsteadiness. Traditionally, the clinical assessment of balance by nurses involves a careful observation of the patient performing selected tasks, such as standing upright and still with eyes closed or standing on one leg. The analysis of balance is complex and involves use of stationary force plates which measure kinetics and may also include video analysis. The standard of care requires older adult patients with gait or balance impairment to be referred to an occupational or physical therapist and/or a specialist for appropriate therapy (AGS/BGS, 2011).

Determining Presence of a Balance Impairment and Referral to an Occupational or Physical Therapist

As the professional nurse observes the patient during routine activities of daily living, she may independently determine that the patient's balance is normal. Sitting balance can be determined with the patient sitting on the edge of the bed or in a chair that does not have arm rests. If the patient begins to lean to one side or to fall backwards (unsupported), there is indication of balance impairment. Such a finding would prompt the nurse to refer the patient for a more formal assessment by a trained physical or occupational therapist.

Additional information including a video on balance assessment can be located at the National VA Patient Safety Center, under the falls tool kit at www.patientsafety.va.gov/professionals/onthejob/falls.asp. A handbook for balance assessment is also provided on this website.

Modifications in the assessment to ensure patient safety

As the nurse discovers balance impairment, it is very important that safety measures are implemented immediately, so that a fall can be potentially averted. One modification in the assessment is the presence of two examiners standing on either side of the patient as standing and walking balance is assessed. For the seated patient, use of a lap belt can help along with pillow props should the patient have poor sitting balance while sitting upright in a straight-backed chair. Careful observation of the patient's position in the chair and their ability to sit straight up can detect a sitting balance abnormality. Use of pillow props can assist with positioning the patient so that they are not tilting in the chair or tilting the chair over towards the ground. Accidental or environmental falls occur when the patient tilts in the chair or tilts the chair to one side or another. Incidents have also occurred when the chair is too small to accommodate the patient. The patient may slide off the seat to the ground, or they may experience muscular pain as a result of the body's misalignment in the chair. When misalignment is not corrected, discomfort and pain can lead to restlessness or agitation.

Static standing balance is best assessed by the single leg stance test (Bohannon, 1984). In this test, the patient is asked to stand on one leg for 10 seconds. If performed correctly, there are no significant balance problems. Because of medical conditions, however, the patient may not be medically stable enough to perform this test without assistance. The modified single leg stance test is then a preferred test to assess balance. Here the patient stands behind the back of a straight back chair and while using their fingertips for light support, slowly lifts one leg for 5 seconds, this is then repeated with the other leg. Another test of balance is the Sharpened Romberg Test, which evaluates the patient with eyes opened and then closed while performing three different tasks of balance. Typically the patient is referred to an occupational or physical therapist for this specialized assessment.

The 30-second chair stand test can be administered to assess leg strength and endurance. An instructional video is provided on the CDC STEADI (Stopping

Elderly Accidents, Deaths and Injuries) toolkit website (www.cdc.gov/home-andrecreationalsafety/Falls/steadi/videos.html).

Should an older adult patient over age 65 living in the community demonstrate a balance impairment or unsteadiness, a comprehensive assessment of the fall or a fall evaluation by a trained specialist is warranted (American Geriatrics Society, Falls Prevention, 2011; see Flow Diagram XX or access URL: www.medcats.com/FALLS/frameset.htm).

Assessment of Functional Reach by Trained Occupational and Physical Therapists

Another test which has been used with older adult populations is the functional reach test (Duncan, 1990). The functional reach test measures both forward and lateral balance. It is simple to administer as the patient is asked to extend their arm with 90 degrees of shoulder flexion while the patient is upright and then lean forward or sideways. If the patient can reach more than ten inches they are noted to be at minimal risk for falls. This test, as well as many of the balance tests discussed, is available through review of the instructional videos provided in the STEADI toolkit, available through the CDC website at www.cdc.gov/homeandrecreationalsafety/Falls/steadi/videos.html.

Cognitive Assessment: The Patient at Risk for or with Changed Mental Status

Assessment of mental status is defined as a "structured examination of the patient's behavioral and cognitive functioning" (Martin, 1990). Cognitive assessment includes the patient's ability to understand and process information as measured by their ability to speak, think and perceive, recall, add, subtract and draw diagrams, judge/reason, and be alert and oriented to their surroundings. For behavior, the examiner notes appearance, general behavior, affect, and mood (Martin, 1990). Although nurses observe many of the aspects of the mental status examination on a regular basis when interacting with patients, the mental status examination requires some basic training on what to observe, on how to administer a mental status test, how to interpret the findings, and most importantly, how to integrate the updated findings into the current plan of care. It is important to note that patients of all ages can develop alterations in mental status or cognitive impairment, owing to new onset of an acute illness or a new medication.

Determining if a change in mental status has occurred

Traditionally, nurses will know objectively and intuitively if their patient has developed a change in mental status. But conversation with the patient is often not enough. Simple, once-answered questions like 'What is today's date?' can suddenly become inaccurate, but this does not mean a mental status change occurred. It could be the patient just did not hear the question correctly or they were distracted and not paying attention, thus responding inappropriately. Other signs, such as slowed, delayed, or the absent responses, can also occur for extraneous reasons. The patient's appearance and behavior is very important to note: do they appear dazed or stunned, or have slurred speech? These may be more indicative of an acute mental status change, but until other objective measures are instituted, a mental status determination cannot be made with complete certainty or accuracy. Objective measures must be administered to verify a suspected change in mental status.

Useful screening measures for detecting cognitive impairment among all age groups

For adult and older adult populations, the Mini-Mental State Examination or MMSE (Folstein et al., 1983) contains all of the basic parameters to perform a mental status assessment. Many others exist too with various age populations. Whenever using any instrument, it is vital that the tool be adequately valid, reliable, sensitive, and specific. Another useful measure for patients in the acute care setting is the use of the Confusion Assessment Method or CAM. The Hartford Institute for Geriatric Nursing provides a useful resource for nurses to use the CAM (http://consultgerirn.org/uploads/File/Confusion%20 Assessment%20Method%20%28CAM%29.pdf). As noted by Waszynski (2001), the CAM is both sensitive and specific for diagnosing cognitive impairment and has been correlated with findings from the Mini-Mental State Examination.

In the long-term care setting, use of the Brief Interview of Mental Status (BIMS) is recommended. The BIMs is easy for nurses to use, and because of its psychometric properties, it has been incorporated as part of the cognitive assessment performed in the 3.0 Minimum Data Set (Saliba, 2012).

For children, the University of Utah, School of Medicine has produced a website and on-line video tutorial which can help nurses detect an abnormal neurological examination among infants, children, and young adults (see http://library.med.utah.edu/pedineurologicexam/html/home_exam.html).

Learner Outcome 4. Recognize fall-related injuries with a post-fall assessment.

Recognize fall-related injuries that can be detected by a comprehensive post-fall assessment.

Detecting Fall-related Injury on the Post-Fall Physical Examination

Falls produce various types of injuries depending on the nature of the force of the impact sustained by the patient. In their seminal research, the NCPS found that patients incurred subdural tears to the subdura even though head injury was perceived to be minor (Quigley, 2011). Ground level falls are also associated with significant mortality in elderly patients (Spaniolas et al., 2010). These findings speak to the importance of not ignoring an injury even if it appears to be minor. Therefore, any unusual or asymmetric findings on the physical examination or any alteration in the neurological status of the patient should raise suspicion for injury post-fall.

In the foundation information on falls at the beginning of this book, various types of coding schemes for injury are presented according to their severity. Typically nurses will follow facility protocol to determine the type of injury and its severity so that appropriate treatment intervention can be determined. However, depending on the age of the patient and location of the injury, it may be more difficult to determine if an injury has occurred or not. One case example is one in which a patient had reduced mobility attributed to age and/or disease. It was fairly easy for the healthcare provider to assume that the patient's osteoarthritis had worsened, causing painful mobility. The patient forgot that a fall occurred (due to cognitive impairment) and when questioned, remarked, "No, I did not fall!" The practitioner needed to take time to explore this further, by thorough inspection of the patient. In this situation, upon closer examination and inspection of the patient in a hospital gown, a large, but very old ecchymotic area was found surrounding the lower abdomen and groin area. The patient had minimal pain on palpation, but a lot of pain with weight bearing such as walking. As it turns out, the old bruise was very significant and indicated the presence of an untreated pelvic fracture. This case example illustrates the importance of always inspecting the patient closely, not just observing the patient walk.

Special Consideration

The nurse will need to use all physical examination techniques to inspect, palpate, percuss and auscultate various areas of the patient's body to determine the presence of injury. Use of a head-to-toe approach is recommended, and documentation of the findings must be specific to the location and size of the injury.

Inspection for Suspected Post-Fall Injury

Harking back to basic nursing, the nurse is responsible for inspecting the patient's skin for any signs of abnormalities. Inspection is more than just simple observation. If someone inspected the patient earlier in the aforementioned example and not just observed the patient limp when walking, the fracture would have been found immediately. Beginning with the scalp and head and moving down to the toes, inspection should determine the presence or absence of abnormalities potentially indicative of injury.

Besides noting the notorious skin tears associated with falls, bruises to the skin and their color should also be documented. Using a figure of a person (as seen on the incident report form), the nurse must indicate on admission and also on a regular evaluation thereafter the presence or absence of bruises. Old bruises are faded yellow, whereas more recent bruises are green and purple. Other injuries to the skin include abrasions, lacerations, incisions, tears to the skin, and punctures, among others.

While most research has focused on the epidemiology of fractures at the hip, vertebrae, and wrist, less is known about other fracture injuries which account for 40% of total fragility fractures clinically recognized (Ensrud, 2013). Fractures can occur to the skull, face, sternum, ribs, vertebrae, shoulder, hip and upper and lower extremities. The location of the fracture is critical; for instance, its position over an organ could pose greater threat for damage. Risk factors for osteoporotic fractures are listed below.

- ► History of falling
- ► Immobilization
- ► Female
- ► Increased age; typically over age 75
- ► Caucasian
- ► Low body weight
- ► Previous fracture
- ► Rheumatoid arthritis
- ► Alcohol intake (3 or more drinks per day)
- ► Vitamin D deficiency/low calcium intake
- ► Medications: anticoagulants, glucocorticoids (AHRQ, 2012)

Clinical Indicators for Suspected Post-Fall Injury

The classic sings of hip fracture include shortening, internal or external rotation, or acute swelling of the leg, pain with range of motion or weight bearing, bruising, and depending on the type of hip fracture, an alteration in the circulation evidenced by reduced femoral, pedal or posterior tibial pulses.

Either change in physical functioning or mobility can indicate an underlying injury. Alterations in physical functioning include unanticipated changes in gait or mobility, unanticipated use of an assistive device or supporting oneself using furniture while walking. Other signs of injury may include displays of pain, such as the sudden holding of limbs, ribs or hip, or facial grimacing with bodily movement. A patient's complaints of pain should prompt further inspection of the patient for injury. Other signs of physical injury, especially among older adults include unanticipated change in cognitive or mental status.

Head injuries are classified as closed or open. Concussions can occur post-fall when the patient's head comes into contact with a blunt force, such as the floor or headboard when falling from bed. Hematomas form underneath the skull and can be life threatening. Any obvious bruising of the face (black eyes for example) can indicate a facial fracture or other type of injury indicative of a prior head injury. The CDC has produced a pocket guide for clinicians and patients in response to the high prevalence of traumatic brain injury (TBI). Additional information can be found at: www.cdc.gov/ncipc/pub-res/tbi_toolkit/patients/preventing.htm.

Determining if head injury has occurred

In addition to the assessment of the head discussed earlier, the nurse will need to inspect for lacerations, bruises, or bulges of the cranium, and palpate the cranium to determine if any cranial injury has occurred. Careful assessment of cranial nerves is then performed along with a neurological assessment including deep tendon reflexes. Using a pen light, the nurse will examine the pupil's reaction to light and accommodation and note the size in millimeters. Other important aspects of the assessment include the vital signs and blood pressure determination. Careful monitoring of the patient revealing headache, dizziness, or any mental status deterioration including changes in neurological findings warrants brain imaging immediately. Traditionally, neurological signs, level of consciousness, and vital signs will be checked every 15 minutes for up to 4–6 hours or longer, depending on the nature of the injury. Patients are monitored for a post-fall follow up period which may extend to several weeks post injury.

In long-term care, we found that the ambulatory elderly fallers at greatest risk for head injury were those living in assisted living facilities as opposed to those living at skilled nursing facilities and those who used an assistive device for mobility (Gray-Miceli et al., 2013).

Useful Screening Measures

Numerous assessment and screening tools are available for use by nurses and healthcare providers. One risk tool for fracture potential is called the fracture risk assessment tool, or FRAX (World Health Organization). Screening measures available through the CDC include Heads UP, a screening tool for patients, and another for clinicians (see www.cdc.gov/concussion/HeadsUp/) as well as an organizational tool for nurses to assess organizational capacity and for the hospital unit's leadership to detect and manage fall-related injuries. Other important tools developed by the VISN 8, national patient safety center include an educational brochure about the patient's risk for bleeding (see www.patientsafety.va.gov/docs/fallsToolkit/EducationBrochure_Anticoagulants-102407.pdf).

Modifications in the assessment to ensure patient safety

If the examiner suspects head injury, level of consciousness and vital signs including cranial nerve testing must be assessed on a regular basis which will be dependent upon the type and severity of the injury. The patient's underlying medical condition and medical stability will also factor into the clinical decision–making process about monitoring level of consciousness and vital signs. For example, patients with underlying hematological issues such as low platelet count are much more vulnerable to bleed when a fall occurs. Therefore, frequent assessments of blood pressure, pulse oximetry, and level of consciousness are warranted, among other pertinent indicators of bleeding.

Patient safety measures instituted include ensuring a quiet environment, eliminating any garments, devices or obstacles that the patient could further injure themselves with, staying with the patient to provide observation while closely monitoring them, attachment of monitors for additional assessment such as use of the pulse oximetry monitor, and monitors for continuous blood pressure readings.

Summary

The necessary steps required for nurses to conduct a fall-focused physical assessment are clearly identified in this chapter. Findings from this assessment help to accurately assess the patient and assist in the overall monitoring of their health status. The discrete elements of a falls risk assessment and a post-fall assessment are differentiated for the various parameters assessed within the examination (vital signs, vision, hearing, head and neck, pulmonary, cardiovascular, musculoskeletal, abdominal, neurological, and cognitive). Where needed, specialized measures are discussed as they relate to collaboration between nurses and specially trained occupational and physical therapists. Important elements of assessment modification to ensure patient safety have been included in areas where unsafe situations can occur when patients are injured or at risk for injury. Once the physical examination is complete and documented, the nurse can progress to Step 3: Environmental Assessment and Modification.

References and Resources

American Geriatrics Society, British Geriatrics Society & the American Academy of Orthopedic Surgeons Panel on Falls Prevention. (2001). Guidelines for the prevention of falls in older persons. *Journal of the American Geriatrics Society 49*, 664–672.

Agency for Healthcare Research and Quality (AHRQ). (2012). Treatment for osteoporotic fractures: An update. *Clinical Research Summary* (series). Retrieved from http://www.effectivehealthcare.ahrq.gov/ehc/products/160/1048/lbd_clin_fin_to_post.pdf

American Medical Directors Association (AMDA). (1998). *Falls and fall risk in the long-term care setting*. Columbia, MD: AMDA.

Bradley, J., & Davis, K. (2003). Orthostatic hypotension. *American Family Physician*, 68, 2393–2399.

Centers for Disease Control and Prevention (CDC). *STEADI tool kit*. Retrieved from the CDC website: http://www.cdc.gov/homeandrecreationalsafety/Falls/steadi/videos.html

Chen, T. Y., Perontol, C. L., & Edwards, J.D. (2012). Cognitive function as a prospective predictor of falls. *Journals of Gerontology*, 67, 720–728.

Chang, J. T., Morton, S. C., Rubenstein, L. Z., Mojica, W. A., Maglione, M., Suttorp, M.J., ... Shekelle, P. J. (2004). Interventions for the prevention of falls in older adults: Systematic review and meta-analysis of randomized clinical trials. *British Medical Journal*, 328, 680.

Consensus Committee of the American Autonomic Society and the American Academy of Neurology. (1996). Consensus statement on the definition of orthostatic hypotension, pure autonomic failure and multiple system atrophy. *Neurology, 46*, 1470.

Duthie, E., Katz, P., & Malone, M. (Eds.). (2007). *Practice of geriatrics*. Philadelphia, PA: Elsevier Health Sciences.

Ensrud, K. E., Blackwell, T. L., Mangione, C. M., Bowman, P. J., Whooley, M. A., Bauer, D., Schwartz, A. V., Hanlon, J. T., Nevitt, M. C. (2002). Central nervous system-active medications and risk for falls in older women. *Journal of the American Geriatric Society*, 50, 1629–37.

Folstein, M. F., Robbins, L. N., & Helzer, J. E. (1983). The mini-mental state examination. *Archives of General Psychiatry*, 40, 812.

Gallagher, S. (2013). *Implementation guide to the safe patient handling and mobility interprofessional national standards*. Silver Spring, MD: American Nurses Association.

Gray-Miceli, D., Ratcliffe, S. J., Liu, S., Wantland, D., & Johnson, J. (2012). Orthostatic hypotension in older nursing home residents who fall: Are they dizzy? *Clinical Nursing Research*, 21, 64–78.

Gray-Miceli, D., Ratcliffe, S. J., & Thomasson, A. (2013). Ambulatory assisted living fallers at greatest risk for head injury. *Journal of the American Geriatrics Society*, *61*, 1817–1819.

Gray-Miceli, D., Strumpf, N. E., Johnson, J. C., Dragascu, M., & Ratcliffe, S. J. (2006). Psychometric properties of the post-fall index. *Clinical Nursing Research, 15*, 157–176.

Healy, T. C., Peng, C., Haynes, P., McMahon, E., Botler, J., & Gross, L. (2008). The feasibility and effectiveness of translating a matter of balance into a volunteer lay leader model. *Journal of Applied Gerontology, 27*, 34–51.

Inouye, S., van Dyck, C., Alessi, C., Balkin, S., Siegal, A. & Horwitz, R. (1990). Clarifying confusion: The confusion assessment method. *Annals of Internal Medicine, 113*, 941–948.

Inman, V. T., Ralston, H., & Todd, F. (1981). *Human walking*. London, UK: Williams & Wikins.

Jahn, K., Zwergal, A., & Schniepp, R. (2010). Gait disturbances in old age. *Deutsches Arzteblatt International, 107*, 306–316.

Kanis, J. A. on behalf of the World Health Organization Scientific Group. (2007). *Assessment of osteoporosis at the primary health care level* [Technical report]. Sheffield, UK: University of Sheffield.

Kristensen, M. T., Foss, N. B., & Kehlet, H. (2007). Timed "Up and Go" test as a predictor of falls within 6 months after hip fracture surgery. *Physical Therapy, 87,* 24–30.

Ku, E., Lu, Y., Schneider, E., Campese, V. M., & Smith, R. (2011). Prevalence of orthostatic hypotension among very elderly persons with hypertension. *Journal of Clinical Hypertension, 13,* A22.

LeWine, H. (2013, October 31). Balance training seems to prevent falls, injuries in seniors [Web log post]Retrieved from Harvard Heath Blog: http://www.health.harvard.edu/blog/balance-training-seems-to-prevent-falls-injuries-in-seniors-201310316825

Martin, D. C. (1990). The mental status examination. In H. K. Walker, W. D. Hall, & J. W. Hurst (Eds.), *Clinical methods: The history, physical, and laboratory examinations*, 3rd edition. Retrieved from http://www.ncbi.nlm.nih.gov/books/NBK320/

Podsiadlo, D., & Richardson S. (1991). The Timed "Up & Go": A test of balance functional mobility for frail elderly persons. *Journal of the American Geriatrics Society, 39,* 142–148.

Quigley, P., & Goff, L. (2011, March 14–17). Current and emerging innovations to keep patients safe. *American Nurse Today, 6.*

Saliba, D., Buchanan, J., Edelen, M. O., Streim, J., Ouslander, J., Berlowitz, D., & Chodosh, J. (2012). MDS 3.0: Brief interview for mental status. *Journal of the American Medical Directors Association, 13,* 611–617. doi: 10.1016/j.jamda.2012.06.004

Salsabili, H., Bahrpeyma, F., Forogh, B., & Rajabali, S. (2011). Dynamic stability training improves standing balance control in neuropathic patients with type 2 diabetes. *Journal of Rehabilitation Research Development, 48,* 775–86.

Salzman, B. (2010). Gait and balance disorders in older adults. *American Family Physician, 82,* 61–68.

Schoenberger, J. A. (1991). Drug-induced orthostatic hypotension. *Drug Safety, 6,* 402–407.

Spaniolas, K., Cheng, J. D., Gestring, M. L., Sangosanya, A., Stassen, N. A., & Bankey, P. E. (2010, October) Ground level falls are associated with significant mortality in elderly patients. *Journal of Trauma, 69,* 821–825. doi: 10.1097/TA.0b013e3181efc6c6

Stolze, H., Klebe, S., Zechlin, C., Baecker, C., Friege, L., & Deuschl, G. (2004). Falls in frequent neurological diseases-prevalence, risk factors and aetiology. *Journal of Neurology, 251,* 79–84.

Walker, M. L., Austin, A.G., Banke, G. M., Foxx, S. R., Gaetano, L., Gardner, L. A., … Penn, L. (2007). Reference group data for the functional gait assessment. *Physical Therapy, 87,* 1468–1477.

Waszynski, C. (2001, November). The confusion assessment method. In S. Molony (Ed.), *Try this: Best practices in nursing care to older adults.* Hartford Institute for Geriatric Nursing, Issue 13. Retrieved from http://consultgerirn.org/uploads/File/Confusion%20Assessment%20Method%20%28CAM%29.pdf

Helpful Web-based Resources

Falls Tool kit

Agency for Healthcare Research and Quality AHRQ Fall Toolkit. Available on: http://www.ahrq.gov/professionals/systems/long-term-care/resources/facilities/ptsafety/ltcgdintro.html

http://www.patientsafety.va.gov/professionals/onthejob/falls.asp

Assessment of Cognition

Hartford Institute for Geriatric Nursing, Consult Geri RN. Available at: http://consultgerirn.org/uploads/File/Confusion%20Assessment%20Method%20%28CAM%29.pdf.

Assessment of Gait and Balance

Falls Tool Kit. VA National Patient Safety Center.

http://www.patientsafety.va.gov/professionals/onthejob/falls.asp

Centers for Disease Control and Prevention. STEADI (Stopping Elderly Accidents, Deaths and Injuries) Tool kit. Available at: www.cdc.gov/homeandrecreationalsafety/Falls/steadi/about.html

A Matter of Balance is a cognitive behavioral program previously found to be efficacious in a randomized clinical trial (RCT). This is a study examining that finding.

Healy, T. C., Peng, C., Haynes, P., McMahon, E., Botler, J., & Gross, L. (2008). A Matter of balance: The feasibility and effectiveness of translating a matter of balance into a volunteer lay leader model. Journal of Applied Gerontology, 27, 34–51.

National Institutes of Health Senior Health. Balance Problems. Available at: www.nihseniorhealth.gov/balanceproblems/aboutbalanceproblems/01

Assessment of Injury:

Agency for Healthcare Research and Quality. (AHRQ). 2012. Treatment for osteoporotic fractures: An update. Clinical Research Summary (series). Available on: http://www.effectivehealthcare.ahrq.gov/ehc/products/160/1048/lbd_clin_fin_to_post.pdf

Centers for Disease Control and Prevention. Reducing the risk of bone fracture, a review of the research for adults with low bone density. Available at: www.effectivehealthcare.ahrq.gov/lbd.cfm

Centers for Disease Control and Prevention. (2014). Heads Up: Concussion. http://www.cdc.gov/concussion/HeadsUp/

CDC traumatic brain injury. Available on: http://www.cdc.gov/ncipc/pub-res/tbi_toolkit/patients/preventing.htm

Educational Brochure for assessment when using blood thinners. VISN 8, National Patient Safety Center http://www.patientsafety.va.gov/docs/fallsToolkit/EducationBrochure_Anticoagulants-102407.pdf

Faul, M., Xu, L., Wald, M. M. (2010). Traumatic brain injury in the United States: Emergency department visits, hospitalizations, and deaths, 2002-2006. Atlanta (GA): Centers for Disease Control and Prevention. Available on: http://www.cdc.gov/traumticbraininjury/pdf/blue_book.pdf. Accessed October 19, 2012.

Owens, P. L., Russo, A., Spector, W., & Mutter, R. (2006). Emergency department visits for injurious falls among the elderly. Available at: http://www.hcup-us.ahrq.gov/reports/statbriefs/sb80.pdf. HCUP Statistical Briefs #80. October 2009. Rockville, MD: Agency for Health Care Research and Quality.

Pediatric Neurological Exam, University of Utah, School of Medicine. Available at: http://library.med.utah.edu/pedineurologicexam/html/home_exam.html

Step 3. Detecting Environmental Hazards and Modifying the Environment for Patient and Healthcare Worker Safety

Overview

An integral component of determining why a fall occurred in the first place relates to the environment. Using pictorial illustration where appropriate, this chapter discusses some of the more common hazards that threaten both patient and healthcare worker safety. These safety hazards exist both indoors and out, ranging from community homes and walkways to patient bathrooms and devices used for mobility in hospitals. Because these issues are so commonplace, many national professional organizations have dedicated considerable resources to educate the public and healthcare worker. Additionally, due to the frequency of fall hazards coupled with their modifiability, employers and healthcare workers are charged with working together to create a culture of safety for all engaged in the medical or healthcare encounter.

It is standard practice for every practicing nurse and healthcare worker to exert due diligence in eliminating hazards while also educating patients about how to avoid these threats in their environment. Employers must create safe working environments as reflected in ANA's *Safe Patient Handling and Mobility: Interprofessional National Standard*s from the American Nurses Association (ANA, 2013). A balance between a nurse's identification and removal of hazards and patient understanding for avoidance of the hazards whenever possible is critical to promoting a safe environment for the patient.

Undergirding discussion in this chapter are the National Patient Safety Goals for all healthcare facilities and providers, landmark recognition and recommendations of the Institute of Medicine, and nurses who are transforming the environment to achieve the goal of falls prevention.

Each section presents some of the more common environmental hazards with (a) the hazard's evidence-based contribution to patient falls and injury production; (b) important tips to facilitate staff and patient understanding and patient education, and (c) resources for nurses and facilities in their effort to eliminate hazards. Risk hazards in the community will be reviewed first, followed by those in the hospital and long-term care setting.

Broad Public Heath Service Objective: Assuring a Competent Workforce by Diagnosing and Investigating Health Problems in the Community

Learner Outcomes

Upon completion of this chapter, learners will be able to:

1. Identify the necessary elements of a culture of safety for patients and the healthcare workforce;

2. Expand knowledge and understanding of environmental falls and safety hazards, to include:

   2A. Expand knowledge of environmental falls and injury risk factors unique to patient settings; and

   2B. Understand common sources of environmental safety hazards for patients and healthcare workers;

3. Institute proactive measures to reduce environmental hazards, reduce falls and reduce injury risk for each care setting.

Learner Outcome 1. A culture of safety for patients and the healthcare workforce

Identify the necessary elements of a culture of safety for patients and the healthcare workforce.

Safety Culture

Patankar, Brown, Sabin, and Bigda-Peyton (2012, pp. 2–5) have developed a conceptual model called the Safety Culture Pyramid which embraces the dynamic balance between four elements defining safety culture: (1) safety performance, (2) safety climate, (3) safety strategies, and (4) safety values. 'Safety performance' refers to those contributing factors of behavioral traits and systemic opportunities that can be managed to improve organizational safety performance. 'Safety climate' refers to the attitudes and opinions about safety held by people who work in the environment. 'Safety strategies' are identified through organizational leadership, overall mission, and history within the organization. 'Safety values' refer to the underlying values and unquestioned assumptions. These four levels of the pyramid are linked in order to create a state of equilibrium.

According to Patankar, Brown, Sabin, and Bigda-Peyton (2012), safety culture is "a dynamically-balanced, adaptable state resulting from the configuration of values, leadership strategies, and attitudes that collectively impact safety performance at the individual, group and enterprise level" (p. 5).

Within healthcare organizations, various degrees of safety culture exist. According to ANA's safe patient handling and mobility standards (ANA, 2013) establishing a culture of safety requires an emphasis of safety over competing goals (Standard 1). To achieve Standard 1, safe patient handling and mobility (SPHM) and A Culture of Safety recommendations are for employers to: (1) establish a statement of commitment to a culture of safety; (2) establish a non-punitive environment; (3) provide a system for right of refusal; (4) provide safe levels of staffing; and (5) establish a system for communication and collaboration (ANA, 2013, pp. 13–20).

Healthcare workers as engaged partners must too: (1) participate in creating and maintaining a culture of safety; (2) notify the employer of hazards, incidents, near misses and accidents; and (3) use the system to communicate and collaborate relative to identifying best-practice forms of communication that are organization-wide, unit specific, and discipline specific (ANA, 2013, pp. 20–23).

As it relates to the detection of environmental hazards leading to falls and injuries among patients as well as healthcare workers, it is particularly relevant for healthcare organizations to embrace a culture of safety, if they have not done so already. Indicators of safety culture in the practice environment from the top down can be seen through the use of:

- Guiding mission statements that address due diligence, safety culture, and practices,
- Statements of value proposition,
- Performance on readiness surveys,
- Unit level policies and procedures,
- Skills training of the workforce in safety climate at all levels,
- Auditing procedures and quality improvement initiatives which provide opportunities for feedback from all stakeholders, and
- Ongoing educational awareness efforts.

One of the most critical indicators in everyday practice, however, is the absence of extrinsic risk factors for patient falls, and reduced falls and injury rates due to accidental reasons.

This chapter presents common causes of accidental falls due to environmental hazards within the community and in patient settings; most importantly, these causes must be adequately addressed by those facilities that wish to embrace a culture of safety.

Falls at Home: The Community Setting

The CDC estimates that thousands of consumers fall each year, across various age-groups. Many of these falls cause serious injury or are fatal. In 2002, more than 1.6 million individuals visited emergency departments for treatment of injuries due to falls. Of individuals over the age of 65, there were 12,800 reported cases (CDC, 2005). Patients living in the community are especially prone to falls in their environment whether outdoors or in. As a public health response, the CDC has created a safety checklist for home falls prevention which is utilized in this chapter to frame some of the more common falls occurring indoors.

Outdoor Falls

Well-established and older neighborhoods are particularly vulnerable to uneven sidewalks and lack of clear markings between curb and landing surface. For some older Americans travelling these sidewalks, whether or not a fall ensues will largely depend upon multiple factors such as their vision, balance, gait, cognition, and footwear, as well as risk-taking behavior. Ability to recognize a hazard and then navigate around it may become impossible for frail older adults who possess reduced righting reflexes. For this reason, many frail older adults choose to stay indoors until they have appropriate support, such as arm-in-arm assistance from a caregiver when walking to their car.

Space When Parking the Car

While there are many issues with getting into and out of the seat of a car, something important is providing enough distance for the patient's feet between the car door and the curb. If patients are entering and existing on the passenger side and the driver parks too close to the curb, the patient may be unable to bear their weight fully on both feet. As a result, the patient may lose their footing and balance and fall sideways as they attempt to get into or out from the car. Figure 3-1 provides an example of this.

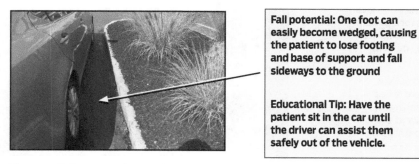

Fall potential: One foot can easily become wedged, causing the patient to lose footing and base of support and fall sideways to the ground

Educational Tip: Have the patient sit in the car until the driver can assist them safely out of the vehicle.

Figure 3-1. Falls potential in a parking space.

Outdoor markings of sidewalks and walkways with bold and bright contrast colors help to distinguish the changes in depth when walking down the steps to the surface landing area.

Learner Outcome 2. Environmental falls and safety hazards

Expand knowledge and understanding about environmental falls and safety hazards to include.

Outcome 2A. Expand knowledge of environmental falls and injury risk factors unique to patient settings

Outcome 2B. Understand common sources of environmental safety hazards for patients and healthcare worker safety

Indoor Falls in the Patient's Home
The Last Step

Inside the patient's home, lighting needs to be adequate especially in hall-ways and corridors where there are uneven surfaces. The illustration provided in Figure 3-2 of the staircase provides a great example of how on a cloudy day without adequate lighting, hallways are dark, posing a safety hazard for older adults. We know that many falls occur on or near staircases. As can be seen, it is difficult to distinguish the last step from the landing surface area, especially when there is no contrast in color.

Fall potential: Dark brown carpeting on steps and landing surface provides no color distinction, thus for a patient with poor vision, the steps blend into the landing surface, easily missed.

Educational tips: 1) Teach patient problem areas and to count steps when ascending or descending; 2) Provide a contrasting color at the base, tacked down to avoid slipping.

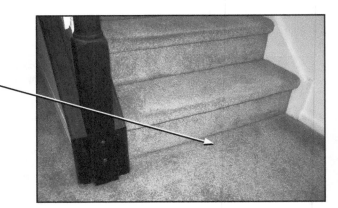

Figure 3-2. Staircase on a cloudy day with inadequate lighting.

Handrails

There should be handrails on both sides of the staircase. Patients who have lower extremity weakness have difficulty ascending steps and may need to hold on with both hands to one handrail in attempt to pull themselves up. In Figure 3-3, the stairs are wide. Frail older adults of small stature may not be able to reach to hold both rails simultaneously (see Chapter 2 on functional reach). There is a potential for falls on these carpeted steps. Depending on the cushioning surface, injury potential may also exist. The nurse should carefully check if the handrail is loose or pulled out from the wall.

Bathroom: Slippery Floors and Throw Rugs

There are many areas of potential safety hazards in the patient's bathroom. Beginning with the tile, floor surfaces can be slippery from moisture or other spills. Often patients place throw rugs in the bathroom, but they do little to

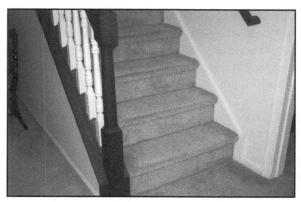

Fall potential: Are handrails sturdy and connected to the wall?

Educational tip: Encourage the patient to report needed repairs.

Figure 3-3 Fall potential of a too-wide staircase.

prevent tripping. Should the patient have a throw rug in a similar color to the floor surface, they may have difficulty in visibly distinguishing the contrast between rug and floor. Figure 3-4 illustrates this point.

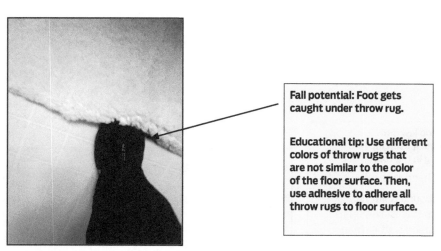

Fall potential: Foot gets caught under throw rug.

Educational tip: Use different colors of throw rugs that are not similar to the color of the floor surface. Then, use adhesive to adhere all throw rugs to floor surface.

Figure 3-4. Bathroom fall potential from hard-to-see throw rug.

Bathroom: Toilet and Tub

In 2008, non-fatal bathroom injuries among person over the age of 15 affected approximately 21.8 million persons, resulting in $67.3 billion in lifetime medical costs. Bathrooms are thus believed to be one of the most hazardous locations in the home. Also, research about the primary body part injured in the bathroom points to the head and neck areas as being affected most often. Bathroom floor surfaces are usually tile and become slippery when wet, creating the potential for a slip leading to a fall. Sharp edges are present on the corners of the sink, while sinks, tubs, and toilets are solid fixtures. When corners and other solid fixtures are unpadded, they create the potential for serious injury should a sudden fall occur. For these reasons and others cited below, bathrooms hazards must be identified and modified.

It is difficult to believe that the illustration below (Figure 3-5) comes from a retirement home. Note that around the toilet there are no grab bars and the toilet height is less than 17 inches (17 inches would be considered a raised toilet, appropriate for an elderly adult). Grab railings and bars add an element of safety for the patient as they can quickly grab them for support. Carpenters can install grab railings directly into the mortar. Pictured here is a plastic bar which provides some assistance, but it is placed too low for when the patient uses the shower, and too high if using the tub.

Safe solutions include the use of a shower chair, where the patient sits to have a shower. In any case, the surface area of the tub should have a shower mat to prevent slipping. Figure 3-5 points to where railings are missing and should be installed. Ideally, the grab bar fit and placement is customized to the patient using it.

Fall potential: Bar is too low if for showering and too high if used for getting up from sitting in the tub.

- ► Lack of raised hand rails
- ► No grab bars around toilet for patient to push themselves up to a standing position (rather than pull themselves up)
- ► Low-rise toilet

Patient and healthcare worker safety tip: Have a carpenter install a higher toilet or purchase a raised toilet seat with grab bars affixed; install grab bars in and around the shower and toilet area; have patient sit to shower and use non-skid rubber water shoes for bathing.

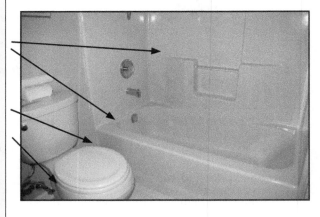

Figure 3-5. Lack of grab bars and hand rails in bathroom.

Grab Bars in the Bathroom

Ideally grab bars are installed customized to each and every patient. Because this is not always possible, portable grab bars can be affixed to the raised toilet seat or side of the tub in the patient's home.

Special Considerations for Patients

An injury potential exists for patients who use the grab bars or hand rails to pull themselves up. Patient and healthcare worker safety tips include:

- ▶ Avoid using a single grab rail to pull oneself up.
- ▶ If the grab rail is not properly mounted to the wall, a serious injury could occur.
- ▶ It is better to use wall-mounted grab rails that fold down and lock when in use.
- ▶ Use grab rails around the toilet that encourage patients to use their biceps and triceps to push themselves up rather than pulling themselves up.

Falls Among Infants, Toddlers and Children in the Home

Unintentional injury due to falls is the leading cause of non-fatal injury among children under age 14 (CDC, 2013). Safety hazards exist even during periods of supervision, and children of all ages are at risk. According to the CDC, infants fall more often from baby walkers or down stairs, while toddlers are more likely to fall from windows. Falls among older age groups are more likely to occur during sports or on the playground. Falls from open windows, down staircases, and from bunk-beds have all been reported by the CDC. Lack of bed rails, staircase gates, and even alarms around the swimming pool can be deadly for children.

Falls from Open Windows

Each year, news headlines include the report of a child's fatal fall from an open window, which often occurs in an urban setting. Typically, parents are home and in some cases, baby sitters are present. Upon careful environmnetal assessment, windows are found to be unlocked, and often to lack screens or security alarms. It only takes a few seconds for an unobserved child to fall from a poorly secured window.

Falls down Staircases

Falls down the staircase commonly occur among infants, toddlers, and children of all ages, and are completely preventable. Recommendations for the prevention of falls down the staircase include use of gates at the top and bottom of the steps. For more information, see www.cdc.gov/healthyhomes/byroom/stairs.html.

Falls in the Tub or Shower

Slips and falls are common in the tub or shower when the floor of the tub is wet. Use of soaps such as bubbles or oils, lack of grab rails, adhesive appliques, or nonskid shoewear, or the inability to sit upright unassisted all pose risks for falls and injury or possible death related to blunt force trauma or drowning. Over 43,000 children nationwide are reportedly seen in the emergency room for tub-related falls. In most cases, the child is supervised. Recommendations include use of non-skid mats in the tub and also outside the tub, among many others. Additional information can be found at www.eurekalert.org/pub_releases/2009-07/nch-sbt070909.php.

Falls from Bunk-Beds

Data collected between 2001–2004 from the National Electronic Injury Surveillance System found that an estimated 23,000 children aged 0–9 years fell from bunk-beds and sustained injuries severe enough to warrant treatment in an emergency department. Most injuries involved the head and neck region. Guard rails are recommended as well as teaching children not to play on the upper bunk or the ladder leading to the upper bunk (Mack, Gilchrist, & Ballesteros, 2007). Additional useful resources and recommendations are avaialbel at www.nationwidechildrens.org/cirp-bunk-bed-safety.

Falls from Baby Walkers

Infants learning to walk often are placed in baby walkers which in essence allows mobility while sitting in a supportive, cushioned seat on wheels. Many falls have occurred when the child encounters steps in the walker. Stair gates and gates with alarms are recommended, in addtion to constant supervsion of the infant.

Hospital and Long-Term Care Setting

Falls in Patient Rooms

Patients admitted to the hospital or those residing in long-term care settings are prone to falls in their environment, such as from beds or chairs. Falls also commonly occur during transfer from bed to chair and vice versa. Based on Oliver's (2010) seminal work in the hospital, we know between 30% and 51% of falls result in some injury and that 80% to 90% are unwitnessed. The majority of these falls occur from beds or bedside chairs with suboptimal height, or when transferring between the two. In mental health facilities, however, falls occur most often while walking. Identified risk factors for these falls and fall-related injuries included a recent fall, muscle weakness, behavioral disturbance, agitation, confusion, urinary incontinence and urinary frequency, prescription of "culprit drugs," as well as orthostatic hypotension.

In the long-term care setting, the work of Becker et al. (2005) found that fall incidence was highest in those elderly frail residents who were able to transfer, but had a recent fall. These findings frame the type of recommendations made during environmental safety rounds.

Bed Safety and Bed Height

There is a body of science around bed safety related to bed height, bed style, mattress type and size, and issues of entrapment and bed falls across all age-groups. The Federal Drug Administration has produced several documents such as *A Guide to Bed Safety, Bed Rails in the Hospital,* and *Nursing Homes and Home Health Care: the Facts* (FDA, 2010), all of which are publically available (see www.fda.gov/MedicalDevices/ProductsandMedicalProcedures/GeneralHospitalDevicesandSupplies/HospitalBeds/ucm123676.htm).

Bed falls can occur when a patient slips out of bed because the wheels on the bed were not locked or not cleaned properly. It is easy for grime to build up on the wheels, causing slipping on a linoleum floor surface. Figure 3-6 shows some common hazards which concern bed falls.

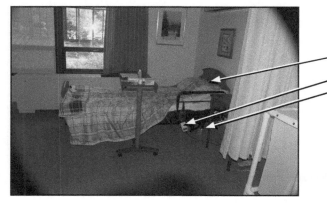

Fall injury potential:
Bed height?
Contact alarm/call bell within reach?
Wheels locked?

Patient and healthcare worker safety tip: Instruct weak and frail patients or those with altered mental status to only transition from bed to chair with assistance.

Figure 3-6. Some common bed falls hazards.

Bed placement within the room is also an important consideration. In the hospital or long-term care setting, beds can be placed against the wall, and when this is done, the patient will need to have a safe exit side from the bed at all times.

Consideration must be given to the biomechanical aspects of patient falls from a bed, as there is a direct relation between head injury and bed height (for additional information see https://www.amemedbeds.com/pdf_files/Spirit/Biomechanical%20Evaluation%20of%20Patient%20Falls%20from%20Bed.pdf). It is recommended that hospitals use the lowest bed height possible.

Falls in the Environment

Floor Surfaces and Eye Glare

Another common issue encountered in practice concerns the tendency for hard floor surfaces to appear shiny or to produce a visible glare. This occurrence can be a distracter in the environment for the patient who is walking. Note in Figure 3-7 the glare production by overhead lights in the environment.

Because of presbyopia, a normal age-related reduction in accommodation of the crystalline lens, reduced depth perception accompanies aging of the eye.

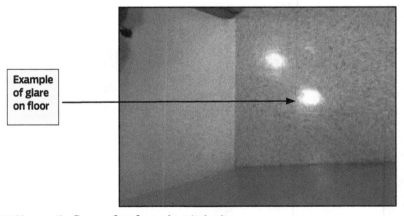

Example of glare on floor

Figure 3-7. Glare on the floor surface from a hospital unit.

Slippery/Wet Floor Surfaces

Falls commonly occur due to spills which make the floor surface wet. Spills may not be seen while walking, especially if the patient or healthcare worker is distracted or if there is also the presence of glare on the floor.

Chairs

Chairs without handrails pose serious issues for getting into or out of a chair safely. For these reasons, chairs without handrails should be avoided all together. In the hospital and long-term care setting, the height of the chair should be assessed relative to the height of the patient using the chair to make sure it is not suboptimal.

Equipment

Bedside Commode

Bedside commodes are used for patients who are unable to walk the distance to the toilet. They may be preferred over bedpans, but do pose their own safety hazards depending on their sturdiness and how they are placed in the environment. In Figure 3-8, the bedside commode has sturdy hand rails, but if placed next to the patient's bed would provide no support and could be toppled over if the patient leans on one arm rail. Proper instruction on how to use the commode is essential, but it should never be used by patients demonstrating weakness. In this situation, assistance will be needed.

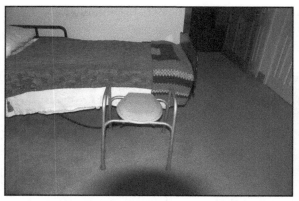

Fall Potential:

Are all 4 legs sturdy, or is it wobbly?

Are broad rubber tips provided on the all four legs of the commode?

Is the commode placed against a supportive structure?

Educational Tips: Instruct the patient to ask for assistance with transferring on and off the commode; stay close by; provide a call bell within reach of the patient.

Figure 3-8. Falls potential of a bedside commode.

Floor Mats

Evidence shows the use of floor mats reduces injury potential during a patient fall. Data from *Biomechanical Evaluation of Injury Severity Associated with Patient Falls from Bed* (Bowers, Lloyd, Lee, Powell-Cope, & Baptiste, 2008) found when no floor mat was used and falls occurred over the top of bedrails, there was approximately a 40% chance of severe head injury. When low-rise beds and no bed rails or floor mat were used, there was a 25% chance of severe head injury. However, when a low bed was used in combination with a floor mat there was about a 1% chance of severe head injury. While floor mats have been used to reduce injury potential and protect the patient from an injurious bed falls in both hospitals and nursing home facilities, recent research suggests that a bevel-edged bedside floor mat is a potential hazard for ambulatory patients, especially those with impaired gaits, using walkers or pushing mobile intravenous stands. In this study, bedside floor mats cause elderly patients with impaired and normal gaits to lose balance, and in some cases, stumble while ambulating onto the floor mat (Doig & Morse, 2010). A guide for selecting the best type of floor mat and other considerations is available through the VISN 8 National Patient Safety Center of Inquiry (see www.patientsafety.va.gov/professionals/onthejob/falls.asp).

Hallways and Door Edges

In the long-term care setting, many floor surfaces are carpeted with a low pile carpet. Between rooms, edging is often present, which can cause trips and falls for patients with decreased step height or decreased vision or those with Parkinson's disease who cannot lift their feet up high. It is very important to assist patients between rooms should they possess these conditions. Figure 3-9 illustrates this situation.

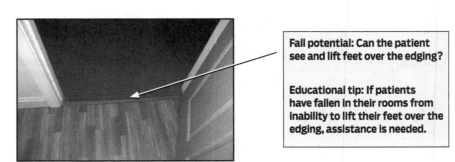

Fall potential: Can the patient see and lift feet over the edging?

Educational tip: If patients have fallen in their rooms from inability to lift their feet over the edging, assistance is needed.

Figure 3-9. Fall potential of room/hallway edges.

Long Hallways in Long-Term Care Settings

In one long-term care facility, the hallways were so long that the facility noted increased patient falls. In order to minimize the environmental accidents, additional seating was provided so that residents could rest. The unit illustrated in Figure 3-10 is the assisted living unit. It provided residents with the ability to safety ambulate by providing low pile carpeting, hand rails, adequate lighting and chairs for resting.

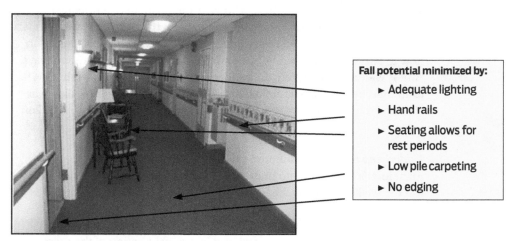

Fall potential minimized by:
- ► Adequate lighting
- ► Hand rails
- ► Seating allows for rest periods
- ► Low pile carpeting
- ► No edging

Figure 3-10. Minimizing falls potential in a long hallway.

Use of Assistive Devices and Equipment
Falls due to canes and walker use

To aid in mobility, residents use straight canes, quad canes, walkers, motorized carts, and wheel chairs, among others. Each of these devices can potentially collapse, have poor grippers on the base of support, or be used incorrectly by patients. The standard of care requires that equipment is in working order and is used properly. Nurses and staff must check the safety of these devices on a regular basis. Many times nurses will work in conjunction with physical therapists to ensure proper function and use of these devices by patients.

The CDC reports more than 47,000 injuries due to falls that involved walkers and canes between 2001 and 2006 among older adults over age 65 (see www.cdc.gov/media/pressrel/2009/r090629.htm). Cane and walker leg tips need to be regularly assessed for tears or cracks. Tips can be purchased or provided by physical or occupational therapy departments.

Mobility aids

Nurses also use aids to assist moving patients. These aids too, need to be reviewed for safety and proper function in addition to ensuring they are used correctly by patients. At times, mobility aids are interchanged. If one does not work for a given patient, another is tried. Consider the example of Mr. P.

> The incident report cited Mr. P., a 90-year-old resident of a nursing home falling repeatedly on the floor when walking on the unit with his stationary walker. He was instructed many times by the nursing staff and family on how to use the walker, but he continued to use it the same way as always. "Mr. P. was observed lifting the walker in the air and walking with it." When examined by the nurse and physical therapist, the stationary walker was changed to a wheeled walker, which Mr. P. now pushes. He has not fallen since.

> *Underlying issue*: Mr. P suffered from recent memory loss due to Alzheimer's disease, so no matter how many times he was instructed to use the walker correctly, he forgot.

> *Special consideration:* The patient's medical stability and underlying medical problems need to be factored into consideration of the most appropriate device to use for mobility.

Adaptive aids

Because of functional impairment of mobility, nurses will often need to use devices to assist with safe transfers of patients between positions (e.g. getting up from bed, transferring from one position to another, etc.). Guidelines provided in *Safe Patient Handling and Mobility: Interprofessional National Standards* (ANA, 2013) recognize the need for employers and healthcare workers to partner to establish, implement, and sustain a formal systematized SPHM program (SPHM Standard 2) for reducing the risk of injuries to both patients and healthcare workers. In addition, the employer and healthcare worker partner to incorporate use of safe patient handling and mobility technology (SPHM Standard 4).

Table 3-1 provides an overview of some of the more commonly used aids and the underlying reasons for their use as illustrated by Quigley & Goff (2011).

TABLE 3-1. **Commonly Used Adaptive Aids.**

Device Name	Utility
Seat buddy ("Lap buddy")	Prevents patient from falling forward if sitting balance is poor; needs to be individually evaluated relative to the patient using the device, as it can be considered a restraint in some situations.
Personalized chair or bed alarm	Alerts the nurse to a change in position or if the patient needs help, but does not prevent a fall.
Smart beds	Beds with technological features (e.g., providing data on the patient, assisting with turning)

The Centers for Medicare and Medicaid have stipulated that if the lap buddy can be removed by the patient, it is not considered a restraining device (see www.aplaceformom.com/blog/2013-8-23-senior-fall-prevention-lap-buddy/). In this case it may be a reminder for patient safety.

Wheelchairs

Wheelchairs are used to transfer patients and often provide the sole source of mobility for patients who have gait or balance impairments, among other illnesses. Wheelchair safety is a concern particularly if patients possess memory loss or cognitive impairment but are ambulatory, as they might get up with the chair brakes unlocked. For this reason, supervision by staff is essential to avert patient falls. Healthcare workers must be trained to lock the brakes of the wheelchair and to regularly inspect the wheelchair for safety. To prevent falls and fall-related injuries, it is critical for employers and healthcare workers to partner to establish an effective system of education and training maintained in accordance with safe patient handling and mobility standards (ANA, 2013; especially SPHM Standard 5).

Learner Outcome 3. Institute proactive measures to reduce environmental hazards, reduce falls, and reduce injury risk for each care setting

Creating a safe environment requires that hazards are identified and proactive measures are taken to eliminate those hazards. One of the first measures is therefore to conduct an environmental safety check. There are several published resources for conducting a safety check of the environment; some are unique to older adults, while others concern all age-groups. Since the incidence of falls and injuries occur among all age-groups and in all types of settings, it is incumbent upon the healthcare workforce to identify and modify these hazards and to educate the consumer/patient about the hazards posed.

Environmental Safety (Outdoors and at Home)

In addition to the home safety checklist provided by the CDC, Rosemary Bakker has developed a comprehensive environmental safety checklist which identifies numerous hazards both outdoors and indoors (Bakker, 2013). As it relates to outdoor safety, walkways, porches, and doors pose significant hazards. The path to the house should be clear and well lit as it relates to side-walks, outdoor lighting, and removal of clutter. Stairs may need repair or there may be a need for a ramp or chair glide for persons unable to climb stairs. As with other rooms in the home, adequate lighting and railings are needed on the porch. Floor surfaces may need repair and can be a scene of an accidental fall. Bakker also recommends that residents be able to open and close the door, and enter and exit the dwelling safely and easily.

Clutter should also be eliminated from the steps and care must be taken to ensure small pets are not lounging on steps where they may not be fully visible. Small pets do pose safety hazards for falls according to the CDC who analyzed data from the National Electronic Injury Surveillance System All Injury Program (NEISS-AIP) for the period 2001–2006. An estimated 86,629 fall injuries associated with cats and dogs occur each year (NCHS, n.d.). Among persons injured, females were 2.1 times more likely to be injured than males (NCHS, n.d.). Recommended prevention strategies should focus on (1) increasing public awareness of pets and pet items as fall hazards and of situations that can lead to fall injuries and (2) obedience training for dogs.

Environmental Safety Checklist in the Home

The CDC has created a safety checklist for home falls prevention which has framed content in this chapter for the more common types of falls occurrences. The following checklist reviews some of the more common indoor hazards (Table 3-2).

Individual-level Falls and Injuries Factors Among Healthcare Workers

There are many individual level factors, in addition to environmental factors within healthcare organizations which influence healthcare worker safety. According to the National Institute for Occupational Safety and Health (NIOSH) as well as the American Nurses Association, healthcare workers are more susceptible to injury when these conditions exist:

- ► Inappropriate footwear (leading to falls)
- ► Fatigue
- ► Poor eyesight
- ► Lack of knowledge or training
- ► Fast work pace
- ► Inadequate nurse staffing

TABLE 3-2. **Check for Safety: A Home Fall Prevention Checklist for Older Adults (CDC, 2005).**

Items within the Home	Questions to ask	Solutions
Floor surfaces	Look at the floor in each room and ask: 1. When you walk through a room, do you have to walk around furniture? 2. Do you have throw rugs on the floor? 3. Are there papers, books, towels, shoes, etc. on the floor? 4. Do you have to walk over or around wires and cords like lamp, telephone or extension cords?	1. Ask someone to move the furniture. 2. Remove the rugs or use double-sided tape or a non-slip backing so the rug won't slip. 3. Pick up things that are on the floor. Always keep objects off the floor. 4. Coil or tape cords and wires next to the wall so you can't trip over them. If needed, have an electrician put in another outlet.
Stairs and steps	Look at the stairs used both inside and outside the home and ask: 1. Are there papers, shoes, books or other objects on the stairs? 2. Are some steps broken or uneven? 3. Do you have only one light switch for your stairs (only at the top or at the bottom of the stairs), or no light at all? 4. Has the stairway light bulb burned out? 5. Is the carpet on the steps loose or torn? 6. Are the handrails loose or broken? Is there a handrail only one side of the stairs?	1. Pick up things on the stairs. Always keep objects off stairs. 2. Fix loose or uneven steps. 3. Have an electrician put in a light switch at the top and bottom of the stairs. You can get light switches that glow. 4. Have a friend or family member change the light bulb. 5. Make sure the carpet is firmly attached to every step, or remove the carpet and attach non-slip rubber threads to the stairs. 6. Fix loose handrails or put in new ones. Make sure handrails are on both sides of the stairs and run the entire length of the stairs.
Kitchen	Look at the kitchen and eating area and ask: 1. Are the things you use often on high shelves? 2. Is your step stool unsteady?	1. Move items in your cabinets. Keep things you use often on lower shelves (at or near waist level). 2. If you must use a step stool, get one with a bar to hold onto. Never use a chair as a step stool.
Bathroom	Look at all the bathrooms, and ask: 1. Is the tub or shower floor slippery? 2. Do you need some support when you get in and out of the tub or up from the toilet?	1. Put a non-slip rubber mat or self-stick strips on the floor of the tub or shower. 2. Have a carpenter put grab bars inside the tub and next to the toilet.
Bedroom	Look at your bedroom and ask: 1. Is the light closest to the bed hard to reach? 2. Is the path from your bed to the bathroom dark?	1. Place a lamp next to the bed where it's easy to reach. 2. Put in a night light so you can see where you're walking. Some night lights go on by themselves after dark.

(continued)

TABLE 3-2. **Check for Safety (continued)**

Other safety tips
Exercise regularly in an individualized tailored exercise program; engage in exercises to maintain stamina, endurance and balance.
Have your doctor or pharmacist look at all medicines you take; some medications can make you dizzy.
Have your vision checked at least once a year by an eye doctor. Poor vision can increase your risk for falling.
Get up slowly after you sit or lie down.
Wear shoes both inside and outside the house. Avoid going barefooted or wearing slippers.
Improve the lighting in your home. Put in brighter bulbs. Florescent bulbs are bright and cost less to use.
It's safest to have uniform lighting in a room. Add lighting to dark areas. Hang lightweight curtains or shades to reduce glare.
Paint a contrasting color on the top edge of all steps so you can see the stairs better. For example, use light color paint on dark wood.
Keep emergency numbers in large print near each phone.
Put a phone near the floor in case you fall and can't get up.
Think about wearing an alarm device that will bring help in case you fall and can't get up.

Training programs should address these areas of susceptibility and promote a culture of safety which addresses staff knowledge, attitudes, and beliefs around falls and injury prevention. A noted component of effective training includes building not only confidence but competency (Standard 5: Safe Patient Handling and Mobility).

Roles and Responsibilities of Nurses and Other Interdisciplinary Team Members in Falls and Injury Prevention

Within healthcare organizations, multiple levels of individuals concerned with falls prevention exist. All levels of leadership and management have a role in the prevention of falls and collectively work together to create a culture of safety. A toolkit for improving the quality of care related to falls prevention in hospitals provides a comprehensive overview of resources for deciding how responsibilities will be assigned in your organization (for more detail see www.ahrq.gov/professionals/systems/hospital/fallpxtoolkit/fallpxtoolkit.pdf, Tools). Tool 4A and 4B are most useful in this capacity. Tool 4A—Assigning Responsibilities for Using Best Practices together with a summary page illustrates how responsibilities might be organized. Nurses and direct care workers as well as physical and occupational therapists who directly interface with the patient assist in falls and injury prevention through the following activities and responsibilities (Table 3-3).

TABLE 3-3. Environmental Hazards and Falls and Injury Prevention.

Role*	Activity*
Licensed Nurse	• Completes and reviews environmental safety checklist and ensures hazards are eliminated; • Educates patient and family caregivers; • Supervises aides; • Supervises the execution of the overall plan of care; • Reports areas of concern to other team members and/or physician; and • Participates in environmental safety rounds.
Nurse's Aide	• Performs hourly safety rounds and reports any safety concerns; • Observes patient and reports any change in the patient's condition to the nurse; • Assists patients as needed according to the plan of care; and • Evaluates the safety of equipment (wheelchairs, beds, adaptive aids) on a regular basis.
Physical/Occupational Therapist	• Evaluates and trains patients in safe mobility and transfers; • Trains and monitors patients on correct use of adaptive aids; • Works with nurses to ensure environmental modifications are completed; • Performs individualized assessments to identify risk factors which are modifiable and monitors the patient progress & communicates directly with other team members; and • Participates in the training of healthcare staff in safe patient handling and mobility.

(* Organized by common roles and activities assumed by nurses and other direct care workers.)

Environmental Rounds in the Healthcare Setting

Walking rounds by staff, as often as every hour, provide an opportunity to assess all aspects of the patient's direct environment: floor surfaces, presence of equipment, use of adaptive aids, lighting, clutter and existence of any active problem areas. Use of a checklist customized to each type of healthcare setting is recommended. During the walking rounds, staff can also observe if patients require additional assistance. For instance, staff may find that a patient is sitting comfortably in a chair or they may find the patient walking without assistance while barefoot. These observations provide important points of additional information which can then be used to frame the overall plan of care and to monitor the safety of the patient.

Environmental Modifications for Patients at High Risk to Injure

Based on information observed in the environmental rounds, modifications in the environment may need to be made in order to prevent serious injury. In general, these modifications will depend on the nurse's observations and assessment of what is effective in preventing falls and what areas need further attention. Environmental modification will vary from patient to patient, and depend on the latest and highest evidence available. Some examples include:

- ► Low-rise bed
- ► Padded bed rails
- ► Use of a floor mat for immobile patients
- ► Scoop mattress
- ► Moving patient closer to the nursing station
- ► Monitoring patients by use of personal alarms

In this context, it is important to consider the VA National Falls Toolkit, which highlights many provider-driven environmental assessment projects and resources. Many home safety tool kits are available, each addressing common features of environmental assessments along with their own unique approach. For additional information see www.patientsafety.va.gov/professionals/onthejob/falls.asp. Highlighted are some exemplars of environmental safety: the AgriLife EXTENSION for improving independence in the home environment and bathroom safety for older people; the Cougar home safety assessment; the Cornell University–GEM environmental assessment; the Home Safety Self-Assessment Tool (HSSAT) developed by the University of Buffalo, Department of Rehabilitation Services; and the Easy Living Falls Prevention Checklist and the Home Safety Checklist by the Minnesota Safety Council, among many others.

Summary

The third step, assessment of the environment for safety, is an integral part of determining the likely cause of the fall by the nurse and interdisciplinary team (Step 4). Many hazards exist both indoors and out and in the healthcare setting, requiring constant surveillance and modifications by healthcare workers as well as consumers. Checklists are a useful resource as they help easily identify high-risk areas and can serve as a reminder for areas that need improvement. Many government agencies and organizations concerned with public safety have made resources available, many of which are used within the public health service sphere.

References and Resources

References

American Nurses Association. (2013). *Safe patient handling and mobility: Interprofessional national standards.* Silver Spring, MD: Author.

Bakker, R. (2013). *Gerontological Environmental Modifications (GEM) environmental assessment: Studio apartment.* Weill Medical College of Cornell University. Retrieved from http://cornellaging.org/gem/enviro_studio_assessment.pdf

Becker, C., Loy, S., Sander, S., Nikolaus, T., Rissmann, U., & Kron, M. (2005). An algorithm to screen long-term care residents at risk for accidental falls. *Aging Clinical Experimental Research, 17,* 186–192.

Bowers, B., Lloyd, J., Lee, W., Powell-Cope, G., & Baptiste, A. (2008). Biomechanical evaluation of injury severity associated with patient falls from bed (CE). *Rehabilitation Nursing Journal, November/December.* Retrieved from http://www.rehabnurse.org/apps/ws_resource/public_index.php

Centers for Disease Control and Prevention. (2005). *CDC check for safety: A home fall prevention checklist for older adults.* Atlanta, GA: Author. Retrieved from http://www.cdc.gov/homeandrecreationalsafety/falls/pubs.html#check

Centers for Disease Control and Prevention. (2013). *Falls among older adults: An overview.* Retrieved from http://www.cdc.gov/homeandrecreationalsafety/falls/adultfalls.html

Doig, A. K., & Morse, J. M. (2010).The hazards of using floor mats as a fall protection device at the bedside. *Journal of Patient Safety, 6,* 68–75.

Federal Drug Administration (2010). *A guide to bed safety, bed rails in the hospital, and nursing homes and home health care: The facts* [Pamphlet]. Retrieved from http://www.fda.gov/MedicalDevices/ProductsandMedicalProcedures/GeneralHospitalDevicesandSupplies/HospitalBeds/ucm123676.htm

Health Indicators Warehouse for National Center for Health Statistics (NCHS). (n.d.). *National electronic injury surveillance system—All injury program (NEISS-AIP).* Retrieved from http://www.healthindicators.gov/Resources/DataSources/NEISS-AIP_88/Profile

Mack, K. A., Gilchrist, J., & Ballesteros, M. F. (2007). Bunk-bed related injuries sustained by young children treated in emergency departments in the United States, 2001-2004. *Injury Prevention, 13,* 137–140.

Oliver, D., Healey, F., & Haines, T. P. (2010). Falls and fall related injuries in hospitals [Abstract]. *Clinics in Geriatric Medicine.* Retrieved from http://www.geriatric.theclinics.com/article/S0749-0690(10)00053-4/abstract

Patankar, M. S., Brown, J. P., Sabin, E. J., & Bigda-Peyton, T. G. (2012). *Safety culture: Building and sustaining a cultural change in aviation and healthcare.* Farnham, UK & Burlington, VT: Ashgate Publishing Ltd.

Quigley, P. & Goff, L. (2011). Current and emerging innovations to keep patients safe. *Special Supplement to American Nurse Today—Best Practices for Falls Reduction: A Practical Guide, 6,* 14–17. Retrieved from http://www.americannursetoday.com/Article.aspx?id=7634&fid=7364

Quigley, P., & James A. Haley Veterans Hospital. (2014). *Bundle of interventions targeting high-risk patients reduces falls and fall-related injuries on medical-surgical units.* Retrieved from http://www.innovations.ahrq.gov/content.aspx?id=2611

Stahl-Wexler, S., O'Neill -D'Amico, C., & Rolston, E. (2011). Creating a culture of safety: Building a sustainable falls-reduction program. *Special Supplement to American Nurse Today—Best Practices for Falls Reduction: A Practical Guide, 6.* Retrieved from http://www.americannursetoday.com/Article.aspx?id=7634&fid=7364

Online Resources

Agency for Healthcare Research and Quality. Improving patient safety in long-term care. Retrieved from www.ahrq.gov/professionals/systems/long-term-care/resources/

American Nurses Association. (2011). *Special Supplement to American Nurse Today—Best Practices for Falls Reduction: A Practical Guide, 6*. Retrieved from http://www.americannursetoday.com/Article.aspx?id=7634&fid=7364

Cameron, I. D., Murray, G. R., Gillespie, L. D., Robertson, M. C., Hill, K. D., Cumming, R.G., & Kerse, N. (2010). *Interventions for preventing falls in older people in nursing care facilities and hospitals*. Retrieved from Cochrane Database of Systematic Reviews: http://www2.cochrane.org/reviews/en/ab005465.html

Centers for Disease Control and Prevention. (n.d). Falls: Older adults. Atlanta, GA: Author. Retrieved from http://www.cdc.gov/HomeandRecreationalSafety/Falls/index.html

Courtney, K.A. (2011). *Implementing post-fall staff huddles*. Doctor of Nursing Practice Capstone Projects. Paper 8. Retrieved from http://www.schlarworks.umass.edu/nursing_dnp_capston/8

Institute for Healthcare Improvement. (2014). *How to improve*. (The Model for Improvement on this site is a framework to guide improvement work.) Retrieved from http://www.ihi.org/IHI/Topics/Improvement/ImprovementMethods/HowToImprove/

Institute for Healthcare Improvement. (n.d.). *IHI Improvement map*. Retrieved from http://www.ihi.org/imap/tool/#Process=3c061d92-9c22-42bb-af04-26ae02ed191c

United States Department of Veterans Affairs. (2010). *Safe patient handling and movement*. (Tools and templates for developing and testing innovations and decreasing risk related to patient handling and movement.) Tampa, FL. Retrieved from www.visn8.va.gov/PatientSafetyCenter/safePtHandling

Bunk-Bed Safety Resources:

http://www.nationwidechildrens.org/cirp-bunk-bed-safety

Bath tub Safety for Children:

http://www.eurekalert.org/pub_releases/2009-07/nch-sbt070909.php

Step 4. Diagnosing and Communicating the Fall Type and Developing an Interprofessional Plan of Care

Overview

Completion of Steps 1, 2, and 3 now position the nurse to deduce, with a reasonable degree of certainty, why a particular fall occurred. Was the patient who fell experiencing an acute medical change in their condition such as an arrhythmia or were other factors associated at play such as an environmental hazard, patient lack of safety awareness, gait or balance impairment due to known fall risk factors or from multifactorial factors? As discussed in Steps 1, 2, and 3 the patient's history of the fall event, physical assessment and environmental assessment should all indicate potential types of falls. Plans of care will not be accurately focused and targeted to likely causes if this determination is missing. Note that the nurse's determination of why a particular fall might have occurred is subject to change, as more and more data unfolds from assessments performed by persons trained in conducting a comprehension fall evaluation and by discussion with the interprofessional team during the post-fall huddle.

Early on in the assessment, the fall may be assumed to be due to a faulty piece of equipment, but as the assessment is narrowed to completion and more data and information are uncovered, it may become apparent that the fall was indeed a result of a modifiable intrinsic risk like orthostatic hypotension. Also, since one single patient can have a variety of fall types, determining one likely cause does not eliminate the possibility that their falls may be a result of two or more distinct reasons or factors. Among older adults, evidence suggests that falls are due to multifactorial reasons (Chang et al., 2004), but unfortunately we have very limited prospective case studies of individual patterns of falls by the same person over time.

Without knowing the exact reasons for all patient falls, the standard of care recommends the use of universal falls and injury precautions for all patients. The standard of care also supports tailored interventions when likely fall causes are revealed (as discussed in the case example later in this chapter).

The goal of history taking (Step 1) is to identify potentially treatable patient symptoms, intrinsic risks to fall, and perceived fall risk factors. The goal of the fall-focused physical examination (Step 2) is to detect modifiable intrinsic risk factors while the goal of Step 3 is to identify preventable extrinsic risk factors. The goal of Step 4 is to identify the likely causes of the fall event and engage patients fully in discussion with providers to develop an overall plan of care.

This chapter will utilize an interprofessional case study approach of an elderly hospitalized patient who is at risk for serious injury, but whose risk factors are modifiable andes could be adjusted to prevent falls. This example underscores how interprofessional teams can work together to reduce fall risk and manage acute conditions to prevent recurrent falls. It also underscores Goal 9 of the National Patient Safety Goals: to reduce the risk of patient and resident harm resulting from falls. Use of the post-fall huddle provides a tangible avenue for communication and interprofessional care planning.

Broad Public Health Service Objectives: Three Community-based Objectives

This chapter has three related public health service objectives:

1. Diagnosing and Investigating Health Problems and Health in the Community
2. Mobilizing Community Partnerships
3. Developing Policies and Plans That Support Individual and Community Health

Learner Outcomes:

At the completion of this chapter, the learner will be able to:

- ▶ Recognize the interrelationship of patient symptoms, physical examination findings, extrinsic risks, and falls and fall-related injuries;
- ▶ Tailor appropriate interdisciplinary interventions to various types of patient falls;

- ► Recognize the value of collaboration with interdisciplinary team members during a post-fall huddle to solve the problem of patient falls; and
- ► Utilize appropriate strategies to maximize effective communication and hand-offs with patients, co-workers and interdisciplinary team members.

Learner Outcome 1. Interrelationships Among Patient Symptoms, Physical Examination, Extrinsic Risks and Falls

Recognize the interrelationships among patient symptoms, physical examination findings, extrinsic risks and falls.

Integrating the Historical Data, Physical Examination Findings and Environmental Assessment

Fall History and Physical Examination Findings Based on Fall Type

The fall history and examination findings provide substantial clues as to what type of fall likely occurred. For some of the more common types of falls encountered, the health history comments from patients and family caregivers along with findings detected on the physical examination are presented in Table 4-1. Rendering a likely diagnosis of the fall type or suspected fall type is complex and often challenging, requiring a comprehensive falls evaluation by a trained specialist. Among older adults, falls are often due to multifactorial reasons. However, reliance on a complete fall history and physical assessment coupled with an environmental evaluation (Steps 1, 2, and 3) covered in this book equip the nurse and clinician to determine potential fall types and what additional multifactorial assessments are warranted.

Learner Outcome 2. Tailor appropriate interdisciplinary interventions to various types of patient falls

Learner Outcome 3. Recognize the value of collaboration with interdisciplinary team members to solve the problem of patient falls

TABLE 4-1. **Likely Fall Types Based on Underlying History and Physical Examination.**

Type of Fall Suspectced by Nurse	Typical Statements Provided by Patients Who Fell	Other Supportive History Provided by Family, Caregiver, or Eye Witness:	Pertinent Physical Examination Findings	Environment
Accidental fall	"I just slipped and lost my footing turning the corner. I knew I should not have worn those high-heels... It happens every time I walk with them."	"She has been accident-prone all her life."	· Normal physical examination · Footwear: inappropriate shoes used for mobility	· Clutter on floors · Poor lighting · Torn carpet · Throw rugs on landing surface
Fall due to environmental issues	"I thought I saw the last step, but the lighting is so poor in here, I must have missed it".	"In the winter, she keeps the shades closed and there is really poor lighting."	· Normal physical examination (no visual impairment)	· Clutter on floors · Poor lighting · Torn carpet · Throw rugs on landing surface
Anticipated physiological fall	"I'm so groggy and confused from that new sleeping pill."	"Dad was fine before the doctor started that new medicine for sleep last week."	· Alterations in level of consciousness suggestive of acute delirium (lethargic); demonstrates difficulty in following one step commands · New gait and balance disturbances (wobbly)	None apparent
Fall due to acute change in condition (Dehydration)	"Every time I stand up I get very dizzy and feel faint, it just started happening recently."	"Since she was admitted here 1 month ago, she has been refusing fluids."	· New onset of orthostatic hypotension (getting up from a seated position or on standing) · Dry mucous membranes · Poor oral intake <800 cc/day · Urine specific gravity high	None apparent

Type of Fall Suspectced by Nurse	Typical Statements Provided by Patients Who Fell	Other Supportive History Provided by Family, Caregiver, or Eye Witness:	Pertinent Physical Examination Findings	Environment
Fall due to chronic disease (osteoarthritis of the knee)	"My knee gives out every morning when I get up, and this knee brace does not help any longer."	"The orthopedic surgeon wanted to do a total knee replacement on Dad 10 years ago."	Presence of musculoskeletal abnormalities (knee effusion or crepitation with range of motion) Limited range of motion of weight bearing joints, enlarged knee joint Gait impairment (limbs with walking) No balance impairment	None apparent
Unanticipated fall due to physiological factor (urge or stress or functional incontinence)	"I developed an urge to go to the bathroom every 10 minutes since hospitalized."	"When I came to visit yesterday evening, she was using the toilet every hour."	Evidence of urinary incontinence on examination	None apparent

Case Study: Hospitalized Elderly Patient

Mrs. W is an 85-year-old female admitted to the medical-surgical unit of a hospital for treatment of dehydration and a recent fall at home. Her complaints on admission to the facility are dizziness and fatigue. Her past medical history includes stable hypertension managed with a diuretic, diabetes mellitus type II managed on diet, peripheral vascular disease and atrial fibrillation managed with 2 milligrams of Coumadin (Warfarin) daily. Her admission laboratory data are all normal except for a white blood cell count of 25,000 and a urinalysis which is positive for nitrates and iron bacteria. Brain imaging in the emergency department was negative for any cerebral strokes or bleeds. X-rays of her legs and hips showed no evidence of fracture.

On admission to the unit she is awake and alert, oriented to person, place and time. Fall risk assessment shows both gait and balance impairment with unsteady gait causing the patient to stay confined to bed on the medical-surgical unit. Vital signs are stable except for a supine blood pressure reading of 90/50 which drops to 60/40 with sitting up.

The pre-injury phase of the fall history reveals this patient to be susceptible to falls, especially injurious ones due to her underlying osteoporosis, use of a blood thinner, and complaints of weakness.

In addition to the nursing assessment, the interdisciplinary team is mobilized to evaluate and treat this patient based on a multidimensional assessment from the disciplines of medicine, pharmacy, and physical and occupational therapy. Their suggestions are presented in the table below (Table 4-2).

TABLE 4-2. **Case Study of Mrs. W: Underlying Factors and Interdisciplinary Interventions for a Fall Due to an Acute Underlying Medical Event.**

Likely underlying factors contributing to fall	Interdisciplinary Intervention
History: symptoms of dizziness, weakness; use of diuretic	**Nursing:** monitor symptoms and vital signs; encourage patient to sit up for 2-3 minutes before standing. Instruct patient to take extra time sitting up. **Physician:** assess intake and output; stop diuretic; add daily electrolytes; encourage oral fluids to 2,000 cc daily; out of bed with arm-in-arm assistance only. **Pharmacist:** Review additional medications used with high risk profiles such as those with side effects of weakness or dizziness.
Physical finding: dehydration, orthostatic hypotension	**Nursing:** encourage oral fluids; start Intake & Output monitoring; assess OH blood pressures every shift, report further drops in OH readings; place patient on continuous BP readings; apply compression stockings to increase venous return; instruct patient to rise slowly.
Physical finding: gait and balance impairment	**Physical therapy:** evaluation for gait; balance assessment; start resistance exercises to increase lower extremity strength; monitor progress closely; once stable, start walking program with arm-in-arm assistance by PT aide; monitor for loss of balance symptoms; assess footwear; evaluate need for a foot orthotic device based on diabetes history.
Laboratory finding: Urinary tract infection and bacteremia	**Physician:** start IV fluids and antibiotic; repeat urinalysis at the end of therapy; repeat complete blood count in 3 days. **Pharmacist:** aide physician in review of medication profile and side effects so that appropriate antibiotics individualized to the patient can be determined.
Potential for head injury post fall (high risk due to osteoporosis history and Coumadin use)	**Physician:** Place patient on neurological checks every 15 minutes for 2 hours; if stable, hourly around the clock; repeat head CT scan; check bleeding and protime levels (PT/PTT).
Potential for additional falls: at risk for injury	**Nursing:** Place on hourly environmental rounds by nursing aides; get low-rise bed; place floor mat next to exit of bed; install a personal alarm; educate the patient of nature of risk and interventions taken.

Outcome of Care for Mrs. W

Within 7 days, Mrs. W showed reduction of her symptoms of dizziness and resolution of her orthostatic hypotension. She began to increase her fluid intake and to follow instructions to rise slowly from bed. As she received IV fluids, her blood pressure normalized. The antibiotic treated the urinary tract infection and results from the repeat urinalysis and complete blood count returned to normal. On the tenth day of her stay, she began to get up with assistance and walk in the unit. She wore rubber heeled shoes and held onto the therapy aide for assistance. Given her improvements she was encouraged to continue PT at home. She did not incur any bed or chair falls, although she was at risk for these events. She was discharged home on day 14 with instructions to undergo a bone oximetry scan to follow up with the primary physician for evaluation and treatment of osteoporosis. She was recommended to use hip protectors.

Interventions for Serious Injury Potential

The use of protective gear, such as helmets, hip protectors, low rise beds, and other interventions such as padding the floor surface, monitoring vital signs, blood glucose levels, serial hemoglobin levels and platelet counts is vital for the prevention of serious injury among older adults who are hospitalized. For head injuries, serial neurological checks and also frequent brain imaging such as CAT scans are necessary, even if prior scans are negative. Careful observation of mental status, behavior and overall function can detect incremental problems related to serious head or extremity injury.

It is vital that agencies and organizations working with patients at high risk for fall-related injury implement practice protocol for treatment intervention. Standing protocol or procedures can help to reduce the high incidence of injuries through early detection and intervention. For example, should any patient fall on the telemetry unit, a CAT scan of the head is immediately ordered and reviewed by the attending physician. Such protocol ensures that additional diagnostic imaging is performed in a timely manner. Nurses should also consult with emerging innovations to keep patients safe (Quigley & Goff, 2011). As illustrated in this case, the use of hip protectors were recommended as well as floor mats.

Hip Protectors

Like other measures designed to reduce the impact of the fall on the person, hip protectors are most often suggested to reduce injury from a potential hip fracture when the patient is at risk for injury. This recommendation is different than earlier recommendations in which hip protectors were implemented routinely for persons solely at risk for falls (VA Patient Safety Tool kit, see www.patientsafety.va.gov/professionals/onthejob/falls.asp). Avoidance of hip fracture is critical, as they are a leading cause of morbidity and mortality among older adults, over age 75. Each year, hundreds of thousands of hip fractures occur in the United States. The clinical effectiveness of hip protectors in actually preventing fracture injury among elderly persons is amongst a growing body of evidence, which varies by population studied (community-dwelling or among nursing home residents). Between the two types of hip protectors manufactured, research suggests that ones with energy-shunting properties are superior to those that are softer with energy absorbing properties (van Schoor, Van Der Veen, Schaap, Smit, & Lips, 2006). This is believed to be due to issues related to human ergonomics behind the way the fall occurs when a hip is fractured. Evidence shows most hip fractures occur due to impact sustained from a lateral fall. In other words, the person fell on their side, as opposed to falling on their back or falling face-forward (Lauritzen, 1996). Some noted annoyances of hip protectors include bulkiness, difficulty of application, and issues of removal when functional impairment exists, among others. All of these circumstances must be factored into the discussion with the patient about use of hip protectors.

Many resources exist to aid the nurse in use of hip protectors should they be implemented among those patients at highest risk for injury. According to recommendations from the VA Department of Health in their National Falls Prevention Toolkit and the AHRQ (www.patientsafety.va.gov/professionals/onthejob/falls.asp) these factors include:

1. (a) Age over 70, and

    (b) at least two risk factors for osteoporosis (smoking, ETOH abuse, malabsorption, hyperthyroidism, hyperparathyroidism, COPD, prolonged use of steroids, antiepileptics, TZDs, diabetes, hypogonadism or total androgen blockade for metastatic prostate ca, female sex, BMI<21, liver disease, s/p organ transplant, etc.), and

    (c) had at least one fall in the prior 12 months; or if no falls, have at least two risk factors for falls (multiple centrally-acting medications such as benzodiazepines, psychotropics, antidepressants, abnormal gait, ADL deficits, impaired vision, peripheral neuropathy, etc.);

    OR

2. Have documented osteoporosis (T score<-2.5) by DEXA scanning;

    OR

3. Prior fall-related fracture injury.

Roles of Team Members in Falls and Injury Prevention

Creating a safety culture requires the input of the interprofessional/interdisciplinary team. Members include nursing and medical staff, pharmacists, family caregivers, nurse managers, team leaders, occupational and physical therapists, dietary members, and all others who interact one on one with the patient. The fall prevention tool kit from the Agency for Healthcare Research and Quality (AHRQ) (Table 4-3) delineates each role these team members have in reducing falls and adverting potential injuries. Recommendations from trained specialists, physicians, and the nurses are best conveyed through the use of post-fall huddles.

Value of Post-Fall Huddles

Post-fall huddles are a process measure to ensure that each patient's fall type is identified and that the plan of care is appropriate for the given type of fall. In the in-patient setting, they are composed of members of the falls team (see Table 4-3 which delineates various roles of the fall team members). Research evidence shows that determining the right intervention requires a multidisciplinary review of treatable causes and modifiable risk factors (Ganz et al, 2013; Oliver, Healey, & Haines, 2010), for which post fall huddles have been successful (Quigley, 2009).

Steps 1, 2, and 3 in this book position the nurse to identify likely underlying factors for the fall in order to determine why the fall occurred in the first place. The analysis provided fosters clinical decision-making by professional nurses. Other team members will concurrently identify likely underlying factors from their respective disciplines. The post-fall huddle provides an opportunity for each team member to present their analysis and recommendation(s) and to finalize an agreed upon plan of care to present to the patient for discussion. Additional detail about conducting post-fall huddles can be found at www.patientsafety.va.gov/professionals/onthejob/falls.asp.

Effective Communication and Handoff for Falls Prevention

Best-practice interventions to promote patient safety always involve communication. If a staff nurse finds an environmental safety hazard and does not report it, it may never get fixed; this does little to prevent a similar fall from reoccurring. Thus, communicating findings through appropriate channels is essential. Use of documentation forms can help, but the key is that staff has appropriate resources and is aware of performance expectations.

TABLE 4-3. **Roles and Responsibilities Among the Interprofessional Team (AHRQ, 2013).**

Team Member Discipline	Role in falls prevention/injury reduction
Nurse	Completes and documents fall risk assessments.
	Monitors progress or changes in medical condition.
	Documents care and prevention practices.
	Reports patient problems to medical provider.
	Obtains consults and medical orders as needed.
	Educates patient and family as appropriate.
	Supervises aides.
	Knows how to obtain needed supplies and/or equipment (e.g., a walker).
Nurse aide	Evaluates the safety of the patient's environment during care tasks.
	Performs appropriate care plan tasks.
	Reports task completion to the nurse.
	Reports any changes in the patient's condition to the nurse.
Medical Provider	Reviews need for specific types of rehabilitation therapy.
	Writes orders for specific interventions, including activity orders.
	Reviews medications for fall risk and makes changes to medications as needed.
Pharmacist	Reviews medication list of patients at high risk based on medication profile.
	Suggests alternative medications or dosing regimen to medical provider.
Physical or occupational therapist	Provides skilled therapy to patient to improve ability to perform activities of daily living, such as ambulation and transfers or bathing and dressing.
	Makes recommendations for assistive devices or adaptive equipment.
	Trains patient in safe use of assistive devices or adaptive equipment.
	Reviews appropriateness of activity orders and asks medical provider to treating medical provider.

The Joint Commission notes communication errors to be common among the underlying root causes for patient falls (see Table 1-7). Even in the best circumstances, barriers to effective communication exist. In the healthcare setting for instance, if the patient intercom system fails, what happens then? Does the unit have a backup plan? Is a chain of communication followed? What happens if that communication is breached? Does staff receive merit raises for performance including regular communication? Does staff work together and in harmony with other departments and professionals?

Effective communication handoff is essential to keep all stakeholders informed and up to date on current events. This involves communication within departments and between departments. Communication issues were a common root cause for falls-related sentinel events in hospitals according to ECRI Institute for Falls Prevention. In fact, more than 60% of institutions who reported a fatal or injurious fall to the Joint Commission cited inadequate caregiver communication as the root cause of the accident (ECRI Institute Falls Prevention). Specific concerns included "failure to communicate information during nursing report, shift changes, or a transfer from a hospital to a nursing home; caregivers not documenting changes in conditions in the medical records; and families' inadequate communication about conditions and history of falling." ECRI recommendations include the use of a handoff communication checklist for shift changes that includes communicating information about the patient's most current falls risk assessment to staff on the next shift.

Another common area of concern is the discrepancy between the written fall prevention care plan and what is actually enacted by staff. Here there is always the potential for miscommunication. Since patient circumstances change from moment to moment, so do care plans. Without follow up and timely communication, errors can result. Incorporating strategies to ensure effective communication handoff are vital. For instance, use of the electronic medical record helps ensure legibility of treatment protocol.

Seven components of effective communication are recognized (Mind Tools, 2014). Communication is to be:

1. Clear
2. Concise
3. Concrete
4. Correct
5. Coherent
6. Complete
7. Courteous

Reducing Barriers Impacting Effective Communication

Barriers which impact on the success of effective communication have been cited by many organizations concerned with patient safety. Some common issues, provided by TeamSTEPPS are outlined in Table 4-4.

In any health care environment, in order to provide safe, effective, and efficient care, all of these barriers must be addressed and then eliminated. Methods and measures used seek to provide harmonization between utilization of time, staff responsiveness and role clarity, effective communication styles, information sharing, coordination, monitoring and evaluation.

TABLE 4-4. **Some Barriers Impacting on Effective Communication (Adapted from Team STEPPS, 2006).**

Lack of time	Lack of information sharing
Staff defensiveness	Conventional thinking
Varying styles of communication	Lack of coordination and follow up
Lack of role clarity	

One way to minimize errors in verbal communication is to write down communications. As it relates to falls and injury prevention, the use of treatment protocol can help relay a clear message about the patient's current functional ability and what they are capable of performing. In order to reduce a potential barrier to effective communication, information must be shared among various staff members. Horizontal sharing of information occurs by word of mouth, where information is exchanged verbally, often referring to a specific care plan or assessment check list. Use of proper documentation tools that refer to the original message is critical, as information communicated can be forgotten or misinterpreted, or can change over time. When there is lack of time, and lack of role clarity, information sharing can be lost, leading to errors in care delivery. Vertical sharing of information also must be addressed so that important feedback from bedside caregivers to the supervising nurse and clinician can occur.

Treatment Protocols

On admission to the unit or to the facility, hospital and long-term care patients are assessed for their ability to function, using standard of care measures to assess functional ability. Should the patient be deemed unsafe to independently care for themselves in terms of walking, transferring, bathing or toileting, assistance will be needed. To facilitate clear effective communication handoff between staff across 24 hours, it follows best practice to institute nursing and/or provider treatment protocols especially for the patient at risk for falls and injuries. Listed below is a representative sample of nursing-directive or provider-ordered multidimensional treatment protocols for patients at risk to fall.

- ► Out of bed with assistance only
- ► May ambulate on unit with arm in arm assistance
- ► Bed rest, side rails elevated
- ► Initiate daily walking program
- ► Refer to physical therapy for assessment of gait and adaptive aides
- ► Post-fall neurological checks every 2 hours

- ► Post-fall orthostatic hypotension blood pressure readings every day for 3 days
- ► Return to bed at 2 pm daily for rest period

These nursing directives for care, or provider orders, are adopted into the plan of care. It is important to note most recommendations that build the standard of care for treatment protocol will be largely based on the highest level of evidence from empiric studies. However, there are also best-practice approaches that are based on common-sense nursing assessments, rather than empirical evidence. An example is the case of a patient in the medical care setting who is wobbly all of a sudden while walking. Best practice in this situation would indicate arm in arm assistance immediately to avert a fall, even though there may be limited empirical studies on this intervention. For a detailed listing of various types of treatment protocols, reference to evidenced-based materials is vital. Here, protocol will vary depending on the type of fall which occurred (acute fall, or fall due to environmental issues), the practice environment (hospital, home, long-term care facility), the age of the patient and the discipline (nursing, medicine, physical therapy).

In care of older adults, compilation of treatment protocols in regards to falls prevention has been completed and published by the University of Iowa's John A. Hartford Center of Geriatric Nursing Excellence and the Hartford Institute for Geriatric Nursing at New York University (see wanttoknowMore-geriRN.org).

Treatment protocols published in these guidelines, and by other professional societies such as the American Geriatrics Society (2010), and the American Medical Directors Association, are age- specific to older adults and determined according to the grade and the strength of evidence from the literature. Evidence-based treatment protocols produced by the University of Iowa's John A. Hartford Center of Geriatric Nursing Excellence follow a standard scheme where the evidence is critiqued, analyzed, and graded, based on research findings and other evidence, such as guidelines and standards from professional organizations, case reports and expert opinion. The practice recommendations, which become part of a treatment protocol, are assigned an evidence grade based upon the type and strength of evidence from research and other literature. The grading schema used to make recommendations in this evidence-based practice guideline includes:

- ► A1 = Evidence from well-designed meta-analysis or well-done systematic review with results that consistently support a specific action (e.g., assessment, intervention, or treatment)
- ► A2 = Evidence from one or more randomized controlled trials with consistent results

- ▶ B1 = Evidence from high quality evidence-based practice guidelines
- ▶ B2 = Evidence from one or more quasi-experimental studies with consistent results
- ▶ C1 = Evidence from observational studies with consistent results (e.g., correlational, descriptive studies)
- ▶ C2 = Inconsistent evidence from observational studies or controlled trials
- ▶ D = Evidence only from expert opinion, multiple case reports, or national consensus reports

Team STEPPS: Strategies and Tools to Enhance Performance and Patient Safety

The Agency for Healthcare Research and Quality (AHRQ) has developed an effective, evidenced based framework and team strategy to enhance patient safety and performance, in the workplace called Team STEPPS (AHRQ, 2006). Team STEPPS is comprised of four teachable and learnable skills: leadership, situation monitoring, mutual support, and communication. Each of these four components interacts in dynamic relationships to influence performance, knowledge and attitudes.

In the Team STEPPS process for communication, a technique for conveying critical information requiring immediate attention and action is called *SBAR*. SBAR (situation, background, assessment and recommendation) has similarities with the problem-oriented record described in Chapter 1. As it relates to patient falls, SBAR relates to:

S: *Situation*: What is going on with the patient?

"Mrs. Smith is on the floor again."

B: *Background*: What is the clinical context?

"Mrs. Smith recently fell and fractured her right hip."

A: *Assessment:*

"It appears Mrs. Smith got out of bed unassisted. She says she has frequent urination from the IV and could not wait for the nurse."

R: *Recommendation:*

"Patient needs to be toileted regularly."

"Patient needs to be toileted every hour, not every 2 hours."

Another important aspect of communication using Team STEPPS is the use of check-back. Check-back is described as the process of employing closed loop communication to ensure the information was conveyed and understood correctly. It allows for immediate feedback and confirmation between two individuals.

> *Example*: Toilet every hour, correct?

> *Response*: That's correct, every hour.

The use of check-backs can assist in ensuring correct communication has taken place.

Handoffs

Handoffs are commonly used in nursing practice to transfer information during changes of shift, but in nursing, handoffs are called patient reports. These reports provide the oncoming shift of nurses with knowledge of a patient's current situation. It is usually during walking rounds that this handoff of information occurs. Patient reports provide an opportunity for verification and clarification of information if needed. They are also vital during change of shift and when patients are transported from one area to another and whenever there is a change in the clinician or provider.

Even though nurses do walking rounds, use appropriate tools to describe patient falls and injuries, and follow communication techniques such as SBAR and handoffs, there are still several barriers to effective communication. Some of the more common of such barriers related to a lack of time are listed below (adapted from Team STEPPS, 2006).

- ► Inadequate sharing of information
- ► Staff defensiveness
- ► Conventional styles of thinking
- ► Varying styles of communication
- ► Lack of coordination and follow-up
- ► Lack of role clarity

Signage

The use of signage as discussed in the introduction conveys a message of due diligence to promote a safe environment. Stickers, posters and other signs are available for use in healthcare facilities. Many of these tools are made available to health providers through patient safety tool kits available from the Joint Commission for Accreditation of Health Organization, Emergency Care Research Institute (ECRI) and Agency for Healthcare Research and Quality (AHRQ). Signage is part of the overall culture of safety which needs to be carefully incorporated into the overall mission and goals for falls and injury prevention at the facility. However, signage that becomes unrecognizable or simple "wallpaper" does nothing to proactively prevent falls.

Walking Rounds

Walking rounds by nurses are an ideal way to both communicate the 24-hour report about patient care on the unit as well as provide an opportunity to directly observe patients firsthand. Every attempt should be made to shift practice away from taking a verbal report from a tape-recorded message behind a closed door and toward ensured patient safety through direct observation.

Patient and Environmental Safety Checks

The CDC provides an environmental checklist which can be used in many facilities. It is available as part of the falls toolkit (see the CDC web-based resources). Traditionally staff will be assigned to perform the patient and environmental safety checks on a regular basis. This can lead to early identification of problem areas. For instance, we know many falls occur during the change of shift. By beginning the safety checks before change of shift, we aim to reduce falls before they occur. This also provides an opportunity to identify patients in need (for instance need for toileting or for pain medication). Rather than waiting for a patient to use their call bell to notify the nurse they need help, safety checks can identify and anticipate patient needs.

Teamwork, Fall Champions, and Promoting a Culture of Safety

Falls and injury prevention is a team effort, no matter what the setting. Fall "champions" often lead the falls team in a hospital or a nursing home by being appointed by a nurse or administrator or through self-identification. Champions are integral to creating and maintaining proper patient safety measures. They rally other team members in falls and injury prevention due diligence aimed toward patient safety. Champions are spirited and motivate others on the safety team to accomplish the task at hand. As part of the safety team, fall champions participate in the post-fall huddle, which is a gathering of the minds for communicating about why the fall occurred and how similar falls can be prevented. Important findings with each and every fall are discussed, almost like a root cause analysis (RCA) of the fall in action.

A culture of safety evolves from the input of these champion staff, along with the incorporation of the best practices, evidence-based protocol, safe handling protocol, identification of why the fall occurred through identification of types of falls, and the provision of trained and skilled healthcare providers. As pointed out by Stahl-Wexler (2011), building a sustainable falls-reduction program involves creating a culture of safety. The five components of the Magnet Model (ANCC, n.d.) serve as a best-practice framework for creating such change: Components include: (1) transformational leadership, (2) structural empowerment, (3) use of evidence-based practice, (4) disseminating new information to staff, and (5) continuous quality monitoring of empirical outcomes.

AHRQ has developed many safety assessment tools to help staff from various types of practice settings (nursing home, hospital or outpatient agency) identify existing cultures of safety and areas that require strengthening (see the AHRQ, web-based resource at the end of the chapter).

Special consideration: Frontline caregivers, the nurse's aide and staff in direct contact with the patient, are the eyes and ears of what is happening on a moment-to-moment basis. The information they provide is critical to the ongoing falls prevention campaign in the unit. Therefore it is important their voices are recognized. Making sure that nursing aides communicate changes in patient conditions and routine patient concerns are critical to ensuring patient safety. Nurse aides can document information by using flow sheets and checklists and other methods to communicate their firsthand observations.

One of the recommended checklists by AHRQ is HEAR ME (AHRQ, Improving safety in long-term care facilities). Table 4-5 explains this acronym.

TABLE 4-5. **HEAR ME Acronym for Ongoing Falls Prevention.**

Item	Activity	Relation to falls prevention
Hazards in the environment	Rounding; using safety checklist.	Early identification of areas needing repair; removal of obstacles; cleaning of spills; prevention of slips, trips, and falls.
Education of residents	Patient education session using flip chart of standard tools.	Engage patient in dialogue and discussion about measures they can take to prevent falls.
Anticipate resident needs	Ask about hunger, thirst, pain, need to get up or walk, need to urinate; offer bedpan or assistance to toilet regularly.	Prevent unnecessary hunger, thirst, pain, and need to use toilet without assistance; which are often precipitators of falls.
Round frequently	Constant observation of patients.	Early identification of patient needs, circumstances.
Materials and equipment	Assess equipment for sturdiness, working order; attend educational sessions and refresher courses.	Equipment which is unsafe can lead to falls. Staff members require regular continuing education updates in patient safety.
Exercise and ambulation	Engage patients in a regular program of walking and exercise.	Use of Tai Chi or strength training exercise to improve gait or balance impairment has a role in falls prevention.

Falls Management Plan

Environmental safety, review of high risk medications, evaluation and treatment of underlying conditions causing falls (visual, balance or gait impairment, shoe wear, cognitive impairment or mental status change), and ongoing assessment of patients are all equally important aspects of falls prevention. Once an individualized plan of care is developed from this assessment, goals are set, interventions are determined and the plan of care is set into motion, ideally by the interprofessional team. This plan of care is then communicated to all involved. The next step is getting patients involved in their own falls prevention, which will be discussed in Step 5.

Summary

Efforts to reduce falls and related injuries cannot be fully accomplished single-handedly. Because falls are complex and often multifactorial, specialized approaches are needed by multiple disciplines, all operating effectively as one team. Fall reduction and injury prevention are best accomplished when this team evaluates likely causes and solutions together.

References

Agency for Healthcare Research and Quality (AHRQ). (2005). *Advances in patient safety: From research to implementation.* AHRQ Publication No. 05-0021-CD. Rockville, MD: Author.

Agency for Healthcare Research and Quality (AHRQ). (2006, June). *Team STEPPS: Strategies and tools to enhance performance and patient safety.* AHRQ Publication No. 06-0020-2. Rockville, MD: Author.

American Geriatrics Society & British Geriatrics Society. (2011, January). Summary of the updated American Geriatrics Society/British Geriatrics Society clinical practice guideline for prevention of falls in older persons. *Journal of the American Geriatrics Society, 59,* 149–157. Retrieved from http://onlinelibrary.wiley.com/doi/10.1111/j.1532-5415.2010.03234.x/pdf

American Nurses Credentialing Center (ANCC). (n.d.) *Magnet Recognition Program® model.* Retrieved from http://www.nursecredentialing.org/Magnet/ProgramOverview/New-Magnet-Model

Centers for Disease Control and Prevention (CDC). (2009). *Simply put.* Atlanta, GA: Author.

Critical access hospital and hospital national patient safety goals. (2006). Retrieved from http://www.neodevices.com/resources/CR_NationalPatientSafetyGoals.pdf

ECRI Institute. (2006). *Falls prevention strategies in the healthcare setting: Resources and tools.* Plymouth Meeting, PA: Author.

Ganz, D. A., Huang, C., Saliba, D., Shier, V., Berlowitz, D., VanDeusen Lukas, C., . . . Neumann, P. (2013, January). *Preventing falls in hospitals: A toolkit for improving quality of care.* AHRQ Publication No. 13-0015-EF. Rockville, MD: AHRQ. Retrieved from http://www.ahrq.gov/professionals/systems/hospital/fallpxtoolkit/fallpxtoolkit.pdf

Haig, K.M., Sutton, S., & Whittington, J. (2006). SBAR: A shared mental model for improving communication between clinicians. *Joint Commission Journal on Quality and Patient Safety, 32,* 167–175. Retrieved from http://www.1000livesplus.wales.nhs.uk/sitesplus/documents/1011/Whittington_SBAR_JtCommJ_Mar06.pdf

Kaiser Permanente. (n.d.) SBAR technique for communication: A situational briefing model. Retrieved from Institute for Health Improvement (IHI) website: http://www.ihi.org/IHI/Topics/PatientSafety/SafetyGeneral/Tools/SBARTechniqueforCommunicationASituationalBriefingModel.htm

The Joint Commission International Center for Patient Safety. (2005). Strategies to improve hand-off communication: implementing a process to resolve questions. *Joint Commission Perspectives on Patient Safety, 5* (7):, 11-11(1). Available at http://www.jcipatientsafety.org/show.asp?durki=10742&site=184&return=10737 Retrieved from https://ps.mcic.com/appdocs/lps/Strategies%20to%20Improve%20Handoff%20Communication.pdf

The Joint Commission (2006). *Root causes of sentinel events, all categories.* Oakbrook, IL: Author.

Lauritzen, J. B. (1996). Hip fractures: Incidence, risk factors, energy absorption, and prevention. *Bone, 18,* 65S–75S. doi: 10.1016/8756-3282(95)00382-7.PMID8717550

Mind Tools, Ltd. The 7 C's for communication. Available at http://www.Mindtools.com

National Quality Forum (NQF). Safe practices for better health care. Available at: http://www.qualityforum.org/projects/completed/safe_practice

Oliver, D., Healey, F., & Haines, T. (2010). Preventing falls and fall-related injuries in hospitals. *Clinics in Geriatric Medicine, 26,* 645–692.

Quigley, P., Hahm, B., Collazo, S., Gibson, W., Janzen, S., Powell-Cope, G., ... White, S. V. (2009). Reducing serious injury from falls in two veterans' hospital medical-surgical units. *Journal of Nursing Care Quality, 29,* 51–59.

Roy, C. L., Poon, E. G., Karson, A. S., Ladak-Merchant, Z., Johnson, R. E., Maviglia, S. M., Gandhi, T. K. (2005). Patient safety concerns arising from test results that return after hospital discharge. *Annals of Internal Medicine, 143*, 121–128. Retrieved from http://www.psnet.ahrq.gov/resource.aspx?resourceID=2400

van Schoor, N. M., Van Der Veen, A. J., Schaap, L. A., Smit, T. H., Lips, P. (2006). Biomechanical comparison of hard and soft hip protectors, and the influence of soft tissue. *Bone, 39*, 401–407. doi:10.1016/j.bone.2006.01.156. PMID 16546458

Step 5. Informing, Educating, and Empowering Patients

Overview

Patient education for falls prevention is one of the many essential elements related to the prevention of future fall recurrence among patients. Providing knowledge through learning opportunities is an integral component of all patient education, and is contingent upon many interrelated processes and factors. In the healthcare setting for falls prevention, nurses have the opportunity to present to the patient all of the relevant information of the fall, the 4 W's of what happened and why the fall occurred, along with underlying causes so that the patient can not only learn but also participate fully in their plan of care. Engaging patients through teaching about falls prevention not only optimizes their own knowledge about falls and their prevention, but it can facilitate patient-centered care. Among other strategies to educate patients, the teach-back method is an effective interactive process which allows for a continuous loop of communication between a patient and a clinician.

Among the six landmark recommendations for quality in healthcare by the Institute of Medicine is patient-centered care (IOM, 2001). Davis, Schoenbaum, and Audet (2005) note "patient-centered care is a key component... that ensures all patients have access to the kind of care that works for them." Patient education provides a wondrous opportunity not only to present information, but to receive information from the patient about what they understand to be the reality of their fall experience (as discussed briefly in Step 1). Why do patients perceive their fall as important? What are their values, ideas and wishes for falls reduction? All of these questions and more can be asked and answered in patient education sessions.

According to research by the Picker Institute, two of the eight dimensions of patient-centered care include respect for the patient's values, preferences and expressed needs and information and education (Davis, Schoenbaum and Audet (2005). Redman (1998) notes three major purposes of patient education:

1. Attainment of health outcomes shown to be effective by patient education: knowledge, coping and problem solving;

2. Facilitation of patient decision making; and

3. Optimization of patient and family care skills related to health, treatment options, and management of a regimen.

Broad Public Health Services Objective for Step 5: Inform, Educate and Empower People

Learner Outcomes: Upon completion of this chapter, the learner is expected to:

1. Recognize the major factors that influence learning by adult patients;

2. Recognize the core ingredients of a teaching plan to prevent falls among adult patients; and

3. Identify strategies of how to use teach-backs in the overall teaching plan for falls prevention.

Learner Outcome 1: Major factors influencing adult learning

Recognize the major factors that influence learning by adult patients

Patient education includes not only what is taught, but how it is taught. There are many dynamics surrounding the receptivity of information by patients including, among others, the message itself, culture, health literacy, and learning style. For instance is the patient a visual, aural, reading/writing, or a kinesthetic type of learner? (Fleming & Mills, 1992; VARK, 2014) Dubbed VARK™ in 1987, it was first articulated in Fleming & Mills, 1992, and it is now a questionnaire that provides users with a profile of their learning preferences (see www.vark-learn.com/). In addition, the ambience of the healthcare setting may or may not be conducive to learning. Noise or a rushed pace of activity in the environment may be distracters to learning. Another facet of patient education is educating learners with disabilities. Careful educational planning needs to be made for individuals not only with sensory deficits from visual or hearing impairments, but also for those with physical disabilities as a result of their fall injury, such as patients with traumatic brain injuries and those with communication disorders, like aphasia. Some of the more well-known factors influencing the learning needs of older adults are presented in Table 5-1, along with some potential solutions to maximize learning. This table is built on Mauk's taxonomy of learning influences in older adults (2010).

TABLE 5-1. Factors Influencing Learning by Older Adults and Possible Solutions.

Factors Influencing Learning	Possible Solutions to Maximize Learning
Physical impairment: vision	Use large print material, size 14 font or greater; use color contrast with one or two primary colors. Provide adequate lighting or aides for magnification and reading.
Physical impairment: hearing	• Make sure the patient can actually hear your spoken voice; This is critical. • Provide the information in writing or through use of pre-printed materials for hearing impaired learners. • Use assistive listening devices to amplify words and use head phones to minimize distracting background noise which can be amplified by presbycusis (high tone frequency hearing loss of normal aging).
Cognitive impairment: receptivity of information and recall	• Establish early if the patient is able to recall key information or if cognitive impairment exists. • Review the patient's medical record for history of cognitive and/or mental status assessments. • Work with family caregivers and find alternative methods of education.
Psychological issues: stress, anxiety, fear of falling	Establish the learner's readiness to learn: • Does the patient feel stressed? • Is the patient overwhelmed with information presented? • Does the patient possess a fear of falling which may immobilize any action on their part?
Health literacy level	Determine health literacy level using standard techniques such as SMOG (McLaughlin, 1969); this includes analysis of the readability of materials provided to patients.
Learning Style	Use the VARKTM scale to determine if the patient is a visual, aural or kinesthetic type of learner. This analysis will help direct the methods used to communicate information in the educational plan.
Energy level: Timing	Establish the peak time of day where the patient will be the most alert. This is essential for avoiding moments during instruction where the patient dozes off. Because older adults take many medications, some of which are sedating, timing of the patient educational session(s) is critical.
Culture Sensitivity	Use Giger and Davidhizar's (2004) model to identify six cultural phenomena: communication style, personal space issues, social organization, time, environmental control and biologic variations.

Teaching Models Used by Educators to Facilitate Patient Education

The nurse educator must recognize there are many learning theories and models of education used in the health encounter to educate patients. Some models take into account the patient's motivation to learn (motivational interviewing) and readiness to change health behavior based on identified stages of change (transtheoretical model). Others focus on behavioral, social learning theories and self-regulation of behavior based on past experiences, coping ability and illness perception.

One of the most useful models developed in the 1950s was the Health Belief Model, which was later modified by Becker et al. (1974) to address compliance with therapeutic regimens. The model identifies key factors influencing the individual learner as well as modifying factors which influence the perceived threat of illness and perceived benefit of preventive action. This model has important implications for falls prevention as it identifies key factors that impinge on the learner's likelihood of taking the recommended preventive action (Becker et al., 1974). Nola Pender's 1987 Health Promotion Model incorporates individual characteristics of the learner based on their prior experiences and personal factors as well as behavior-specific cognition and affect influencing the individual learner to produce behavior outcomes related to developing a plan of action based on health promotion. An integral prelude to health-promoting behavior is the patient's commitment to an appropriate plan of action (Pender, 1996).

Learner Outcome 2: Recognize the Core ingredients of a falls-prevention teaching plan

Recognize the core ingredients of a teaching plan to prevent falls among adult patients.

Core Ingredients of the Teaching Plan

The elements of a teaching plan include patient goals (short range, intermediate range, and long range), anticipated learner outcomes based on those goals, the actual didactic content delivered, teaching strategies used to deliver the content (recommended in this chapter is the teach-back method), the method of evaluation to assess if learning took place, and lastly any measures used to evaluate the impact of the teaching on the individual patient or community of learners.

If the goal of patient education is to prevent falls from reoccurring, educators must first begin by identifying the message and recognizing how it can be best delivered. Many sources, most notably Simply Put (CDC, 2009), emphasize the simplicity of messaging content. Some of the signage produced by the Centers for Disease Control and Prevention of the Veterans Administration

(CDC and the National Center for Patient Safety [NCPS]) takes into consideration this simplicity for messaging.

Communicating the Fall Message

In creating the fall message for older patients, some considerations recommended by the CDC include: (1) Develop message points—short, concise statements that reflect your main message; (2) Develop themes or adapt materials that will engage patients; (3) Produce materials (computer-generated presentations, flyers, etc.) that will effectively convey your messages; and (4) Pre-test your materials (CDC, 2008).

Evidence shows that the content in the fall prevention message is critical. Because of older adults' perceptions of negative messaging, educators must always focus on the positive and deemphasize age or age-related issues. Some challenges identified by states engaged in fall prevention were identified by stakeholders. Washington reported that "[s]eniors don't tell their health care providers about falls—they are too embarrassed, ashamed, or afraid of losing their independence" (CDC, 2008). What was learned was that messages should be kept positive when educating patients. Based on focus group input from older adults, states found that older adults perceive "falls prevention" as a negative message. Thus, the majority of states interviewed are using positive falls prevention messaging. Example slogans include: "Stay Active and Independent for Life" (Washington), "Catch Yourself: Simple Steps to Prevent Falls" (California), "Keeping Seniors Independent" (New York), and "Keys to Independence" (Massachusetts), among others. Fear-based messaging is often viewed very negatively. Recommendations for appropriate terms are included in Table 5-2.

TABLE 5-2. **Fall Message: Wording to Use or Avoid.**

Some Words and Phrases That Emphasize the Positive	Words and Phrases to Avoid
Independence	Dependent
Staying active	Immobile; inactivity
Moving forward independently	Aging; getting old
Physically active	Fear of falling
Healthy	Illness

Learner Outcome 3: Identify Teach-back strategies in falls prevention teaching

Identify strategies on how to use teach-backs in the teaching plan for falls prevention.

Use of Teach-Backs for Falls Prevention Education

Simply put, teach-back is a way to deliver patient-centered care by focusing patient education on what the patient understands or does not understand. It does not rely on any theory or framework. It allows the patient to openly state what they understand or need clarification about. Teach-backs for falls are dependent on what patients currently understand about their fall, its causes and its prevention.

Patient understanding of the 4 W's of the fall situation—what, when, where, why (described in Chapter 1, page 45)—can be applied in the teach-back model of patient education. A sample conversation may include the following questions: "Today we talked about how falls occur at any age; can you please explain back to me how your fall occurred yesterday while you were walking down the hallway?" "When you are discharged home today, what will you tell your husband about changes needed in your bathroom shower area?" "We talked a lot today about your medications and how some make you drowsy and how the drowsiness caused your fall; in your own words, please tell me what we discussed and what you might do should drowsiness affect you at home?"

Toolkits and videos for using the teach-back method are available. The American Medical Association recommends use of the teach-back method for improving doctor-patient communication (Weiss, 2007).

Steps for Implementing the Teach-Back Method

The teach-back method begins with identifying and remediating factors (that are identified in Table 5-1) that influence patient education prior to the start of the teaching session. After this, the clinician explains any new concept or health information, recommendation(s) and/or changes in management approach. The clinician can use a variety of learning tools at the bedside such as a handheld clipboard, white board, video, closed-caption television, professional charts, diagrams or figures to illustrate concepts. Selection of the appropriate tool will depend on many factors including resources available, content, and message as well as issues related to reliability and validity of the resource, where appropriate. The aides listed above are particularly useful for visual learners. However, kinesthetic learners however learn best with use of tactile methods such as touch or hands-on demonstration at the bedside. Auditory learners learn best by audio recordings, audio books or tape-recorded messages.

Once the information is delivered to the client, the clinician assesses the patient's recall and comprehension, and then clarifies any misconceptions. The clinician then reassesses the patient's recall and comprehension. Nurse researchers have shown that patients who received self-care instructions from nurses using the teach-back method retained significantly more information than those educated with briefer types of teaching methods. The teach-back sessions averaged 34 minutes in length. During hospitalization, 84% of patients answered at least 75% correct and 77% of patients answered correctly on follow-up (White et al., 2013). Retention of health information is an important component to treatment adherence. Xu (2012) offers a wonderful overview of using the teach-back method for patient education and self-management in the American Nurse Today. In her discussion she emphasizes closing the loop of communication and use of the teach-back as a self-management tool to monitor symptoms, adjust medications, incorporate use of exercise into daily routine and identify when to seek medical advice, among other functions.

The teach-back method has been highlighted in many clinical research works to assess comprehension (Kripalani et al., 2008); to quantify and compare clinician's assessments of patient understanding (Farrell et al., 2009) and to increase communication about immunization (Wilson et al., 2008).

Toolkits for using the teach-back method and videos are available through governmental agencies such as AHRQ. The American Medical Association recommends use of the teach-back or "show-me" method as a method for improving doctor-patient communication (Weiss, 2007). Another helpful resource is the North Carolina Program on Health Literacy, where the teach-back method is highlighted (www.nchealthliteracy.org/toolkit/tool5.pdf).

References

Becker, M., Drachman, R., & Kirscht, J. (1974). A new approach to explaining sick-role behavior in low-income populations. *American Journal of Public Health, 64*, 205–216. Retrieved from http://www.ncbi.nlm.nih.gov/pmc/articles/PMC1775416/

Centers for Disease Control and Prevention (CDC). (2008). Preventing falls: How to develop community-based fall prevention programs for older adults. Atlanta, GA: Author.

Centers for Disease Control and Prevention (CDC). (2009). *Simply put: A guide for creating easy-to-understand materials* (3rd ed.). Atlanta, GA: Author.

Davis, K., Schoen, C., & Schoenbaum, S. C. (2000). A 2020 vision of American health care. *Archives of Internalal Medicine, 160*, 3357–62.

Farrell, M. H., Kuruvilla, P., Eskra, K. L., Christopher, S. A., & Brienza, R. S. (2009). A method to quantify and compare clinicians assessments of patient understanding during counseling of standardized patients. *Patient Education Counseling, 77*, 128–35.

Fleming, N. D., & Mills, C. (1992). Not another inventory, rather a catalyst for reflection. *To Improve the Academy, 11*, 137–155.

Giger, J., & Davidhizar, R. (2004). *Transcultural nursing: Assessment and intervention* (5th ed.). St. Louis, MO: Mosby Yearbook, Inc.

Institute of Medicine (IOM). (2001). *Crossing the quality chasm: A new health system for the 21st Century* (Vol. 6). Washington, DC: National Academy Press.

Kripalani, S., Bengtzen, R., Henderson, L. E., & Jacobson, T. A. (2008). Clinical research in low-literacy populations using teach-back to assess comprehension of informed consent and privacy information. *Institutional Review Board, 30*, 13–19.

Mauk, K. L. (2010). *Gerontological nursing: Competencies for care* (2nd ed.). Sudbury, MA: Jones & Bartlett Learning.

McLaughlin, G. H. (1969). SMOG-grading: A new readability formula. *Journal of Reading, 12*, 639–646.

Pender, N. (1996). *Health promotion nursing practice* (3rd ed.), p. 67. Upper Saddle River, NJ: Pearson Education.

Redman, B. K. (1998). *Measurement tools in patient education.* New York: NY. Springer Publications.

Schneider, E. C. (2009). *Falls prevention awareness: Findings and lessons learned from state coalitions on fall prevention.* Washington, DC: National Council on Aging. Available online at www.healthyagingprograms.org.

Weiss, B. D. (2007). *Health literacy and patient safety: Help patients understand. A manual for clinicians* (2nd ed.). Chicago, IL: American Medical Association Foundation and American Medical Association.

White, M., Garbez, R., Carroll, M., Brinker, E., & Howie-Esquivel, J. (2013). Is teach-back associated with knowledge retention and hospital readmission in hospitalized heart failure patients? *Journal of Cardiovascular Nursing, 28*, 137–46. doi:10.1097/JCN.0b013e31824987bd

Wilson, F. L., Baker, L. M., Nordstrom, C. K., & Legwand, C. (2008). Using the teach-back and Orem's Self-care Deficit Nursing theory to increase childhood immunizations communication among low-income mothers. *Issues in Comprehensive Pediatric Nurse, 31*, 7–22.

Xu, P. (2012). Using teach-back for patient education and self-management. *American Nurse Today, 7*, 2.

Index